SIMPLIFIED ARTERIAL

BLOOD GASES

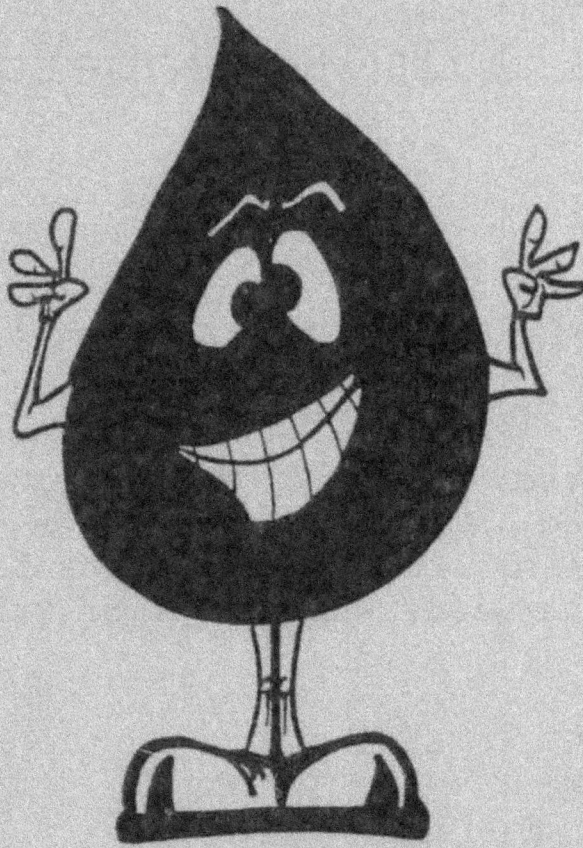

SIMPLIFIED

ARTERIAL

BLOOD GASES

by

Malcolm Rosenberg, R.N.

FOUR EXCELLENT REASONS TO BREATHE

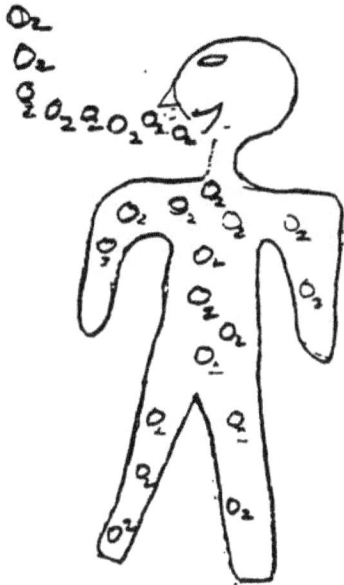

Your body needs oxygen

It needs to get rid of CO_2

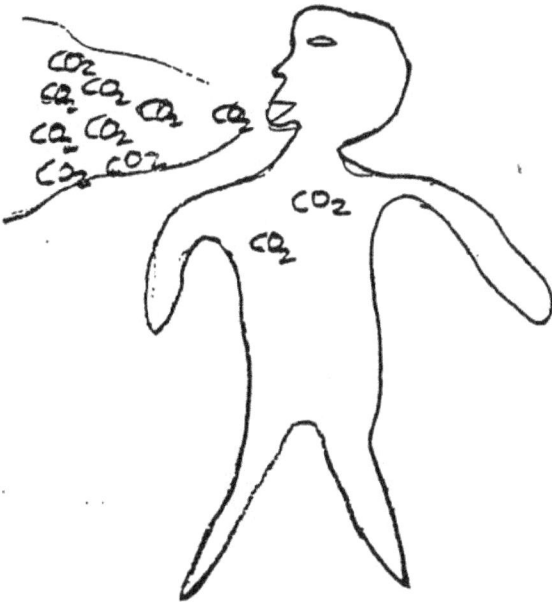

Breathing maintains proper acid levels

It feels good

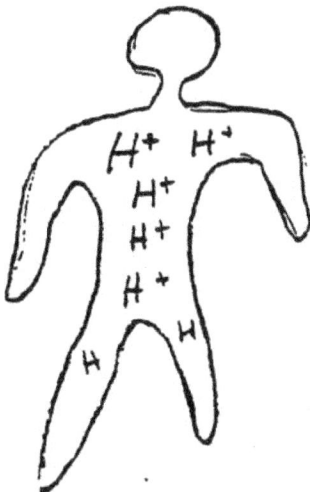

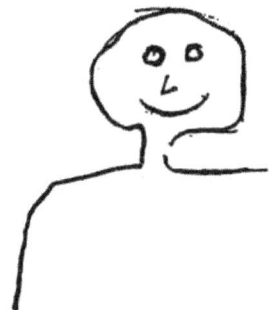

-1-

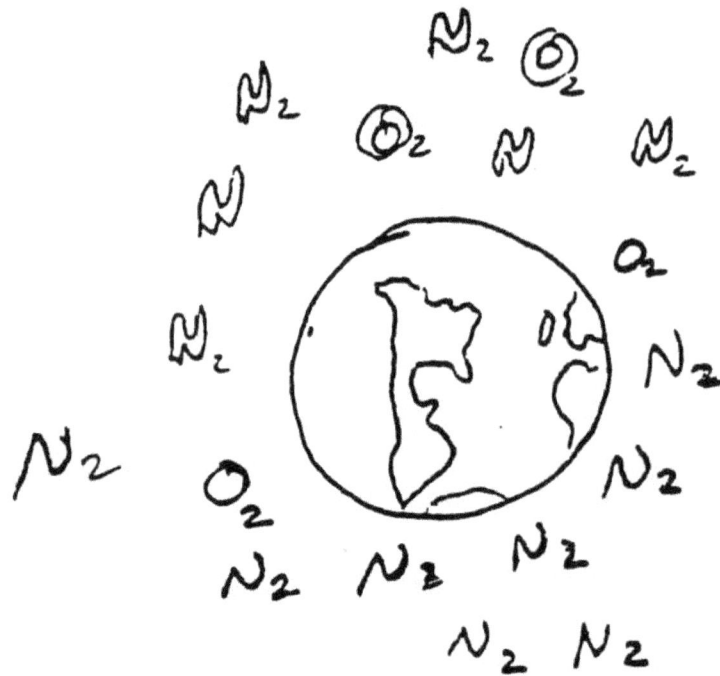

The earth is surrounded by an
atmosphere of gas. Almost all
of it is oxygen (O_2) and nitrogen (N_2).

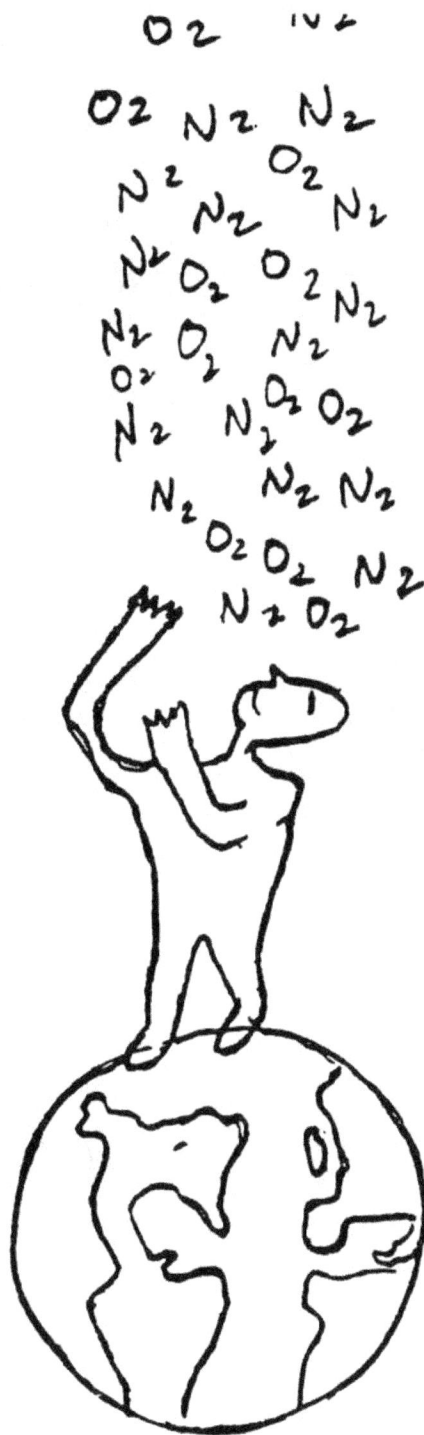

The weight of all that gas in the
atmosphere causes a pressure of
14.7 pounds per square inch.

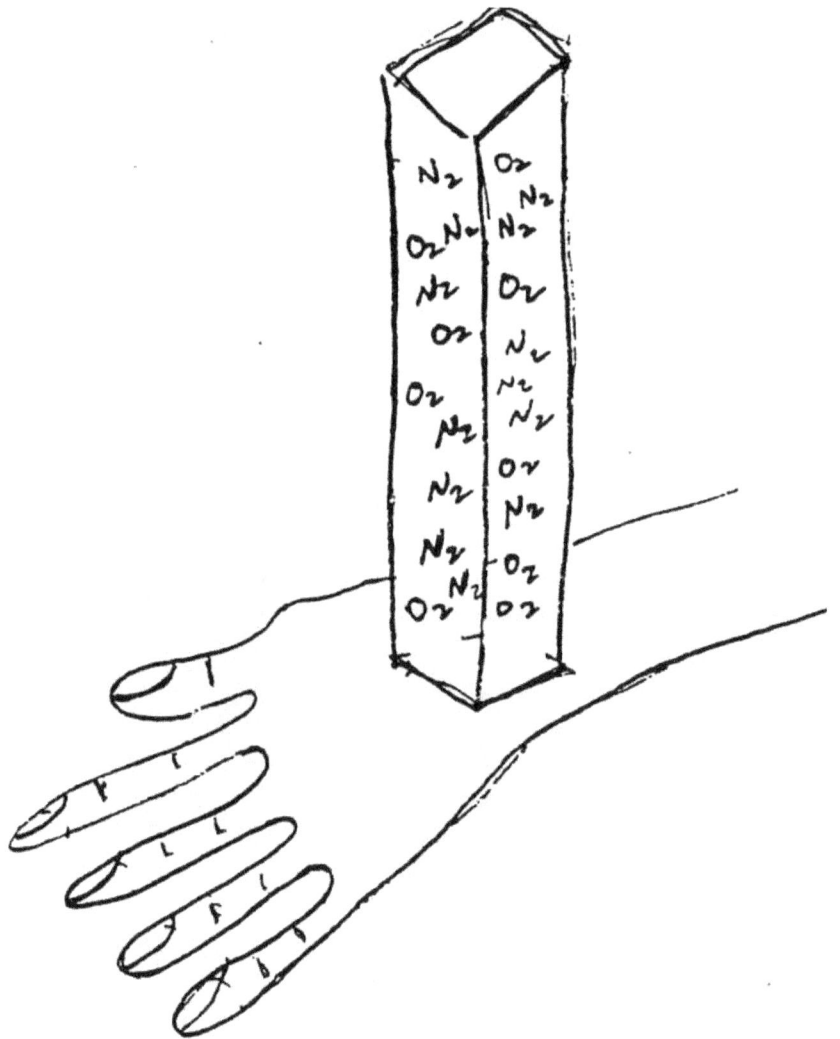

That means the
atmosphere weighs
14.7 pounds on
every square inch
of your body.

14.7 lbs

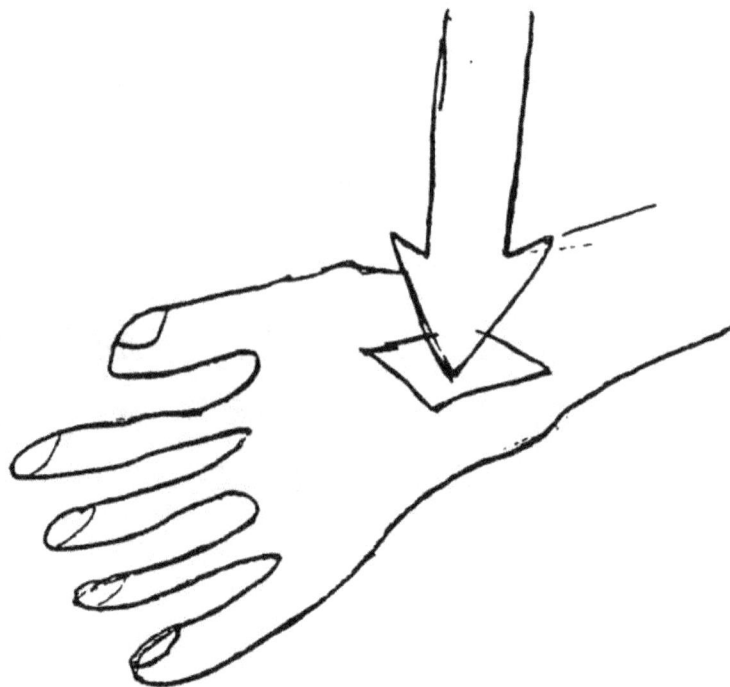

Another way to say pressure is "millimeters
of mercury" or abbreviated "mm Hg." On
weather on television they say "Barometric
pressure is.... millimeters of mercury
today." Millimeters of mercury means how
high a column of mercury (like in a glass
thermometer) would balance the atmospheric
pressure. Normally atmospheric pressure is
760 millimeters (about 30"). In Blood gases
most pressures are stated in "mm Hg."

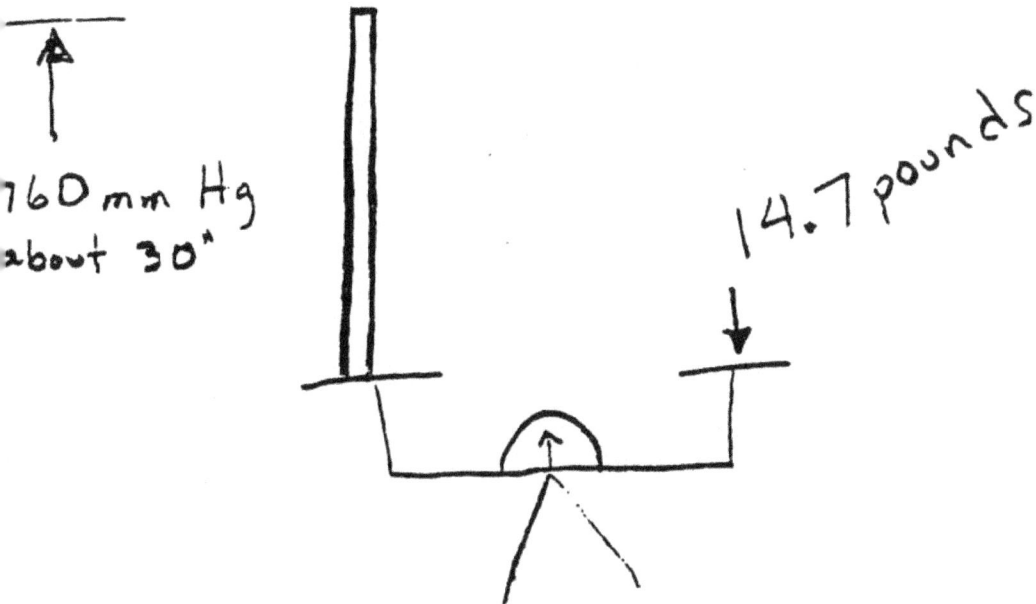

760 mm Hg
about 30"

14.7 pounds

Do you see how the 760mm Hg balances
atmospheric pressure on this scale?

All breathing air in and out of our lungs is working with (on inspiration) and working against (on expiration) that column of air.

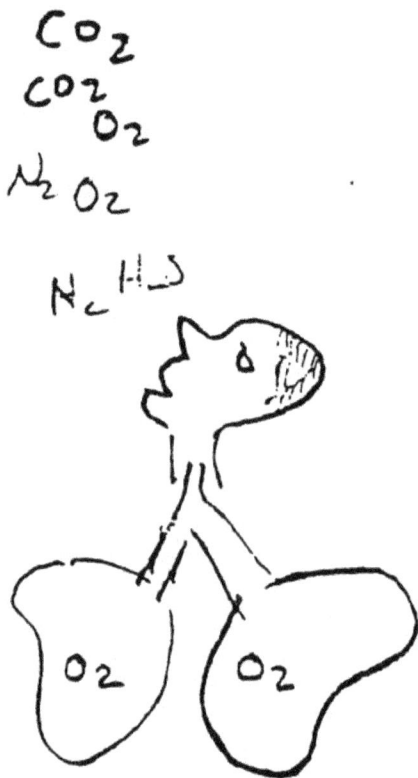

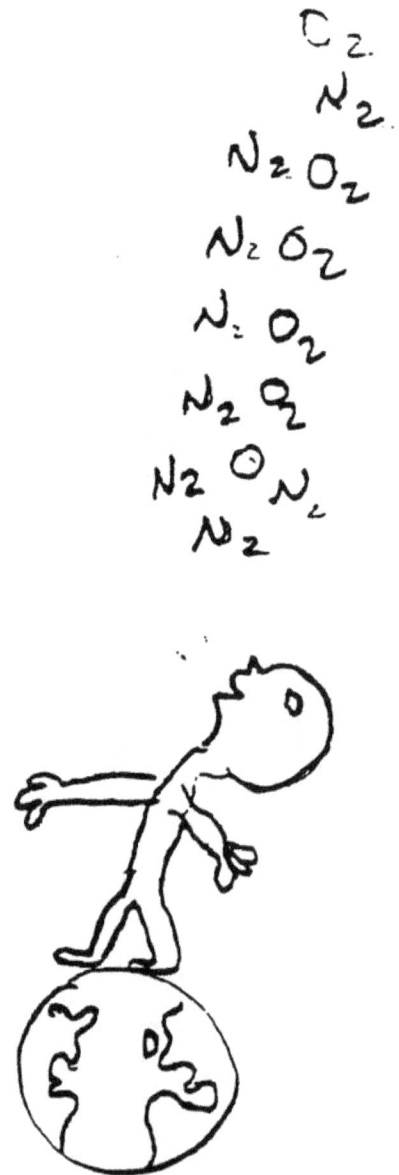

The amount of oxygen that gets into our
blood depends on that pressure. In
Denver which is 3000 feet above sea
level, the column of air causes less

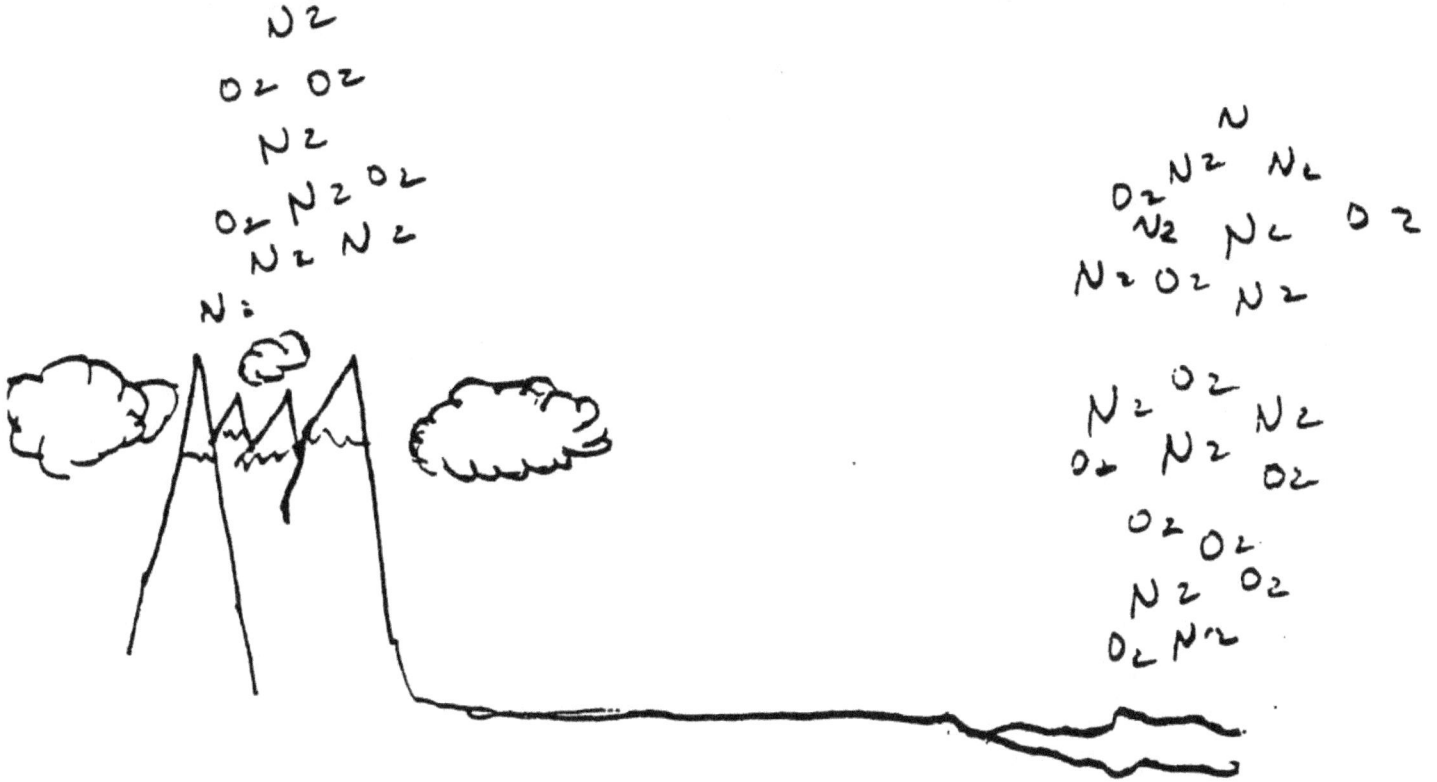

N_2

O_2 O_2

N_2

O_2 N_2 O_2

N_2 N_2

N_2

N

O_2 N_2 N_2

N_2 N_2 O_2

N_2 O_2 N_2

N_2 O_2

N_2 N_2

O_2 N_2 O_2

O_2 O_2

N_2 O_2

O_2 N_2

atmospheric pressure than in Miami.
Maybe that's why the Miami Dolphins
beat the Denver Broncos.

Pressure

You can intuitively understand pressure.

Let's look at some examples.

The pressure you exert by pushing down on something

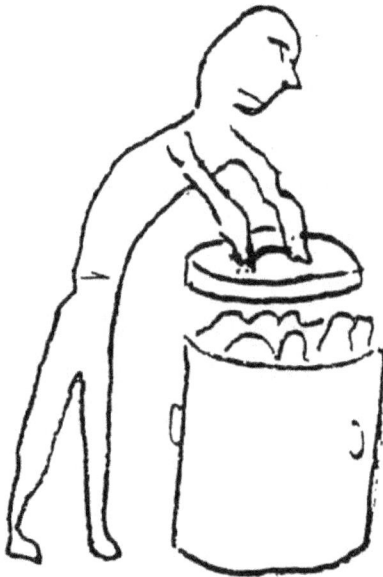

is similar to the pressure the column of air exerts.

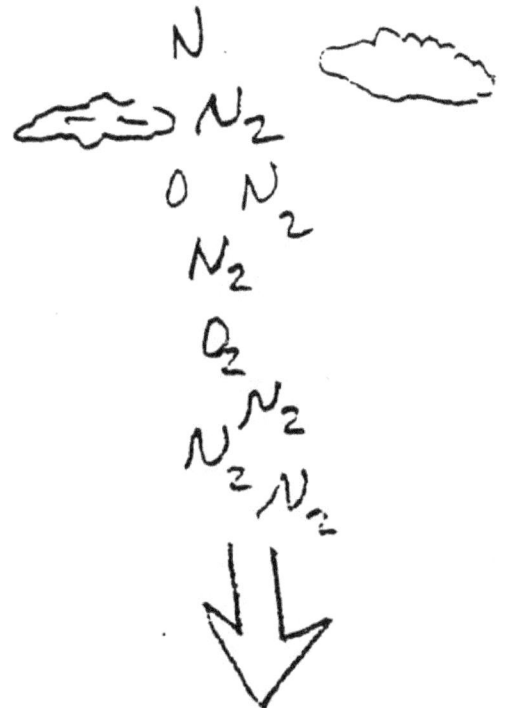

Pressure

The pressure you exert by pushing outward

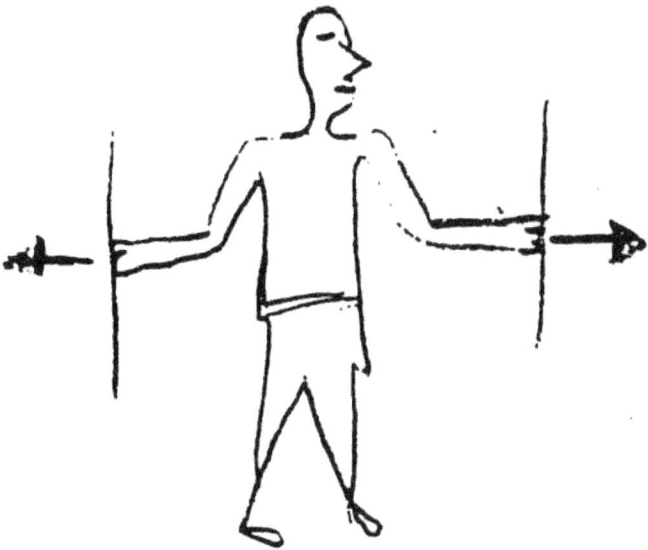

is similar to gas pressure within a closed container.

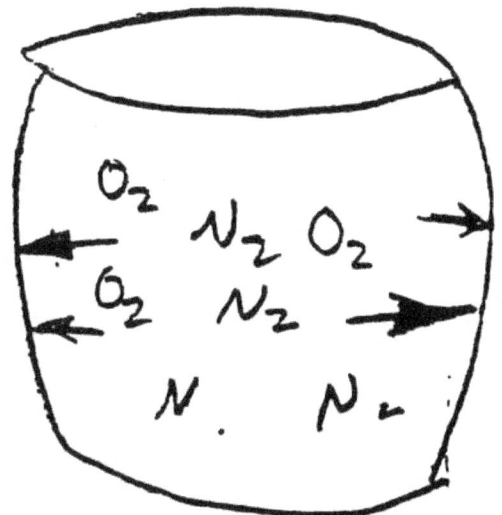

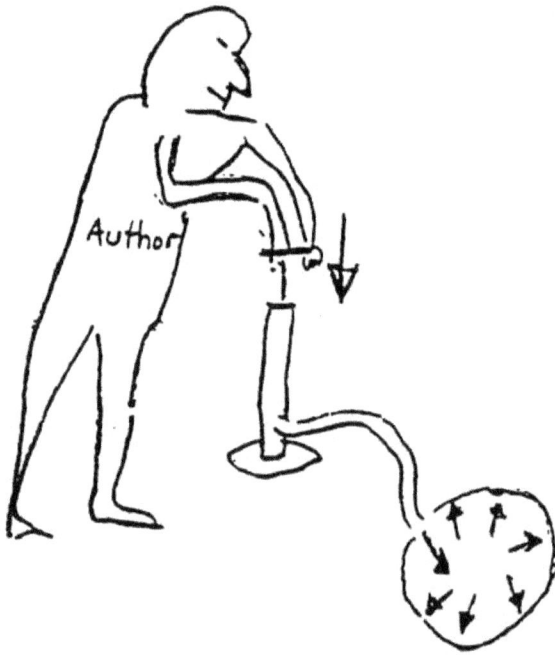

The downward pressure I
exert on a bicycle pump
is transferred to
outward pressure on the
balloon.

That is similar to the atmospheric pressure
expanding your lungs.

N_2
N_2
N_2
N_2
O_2
N_2
O_2
N_2

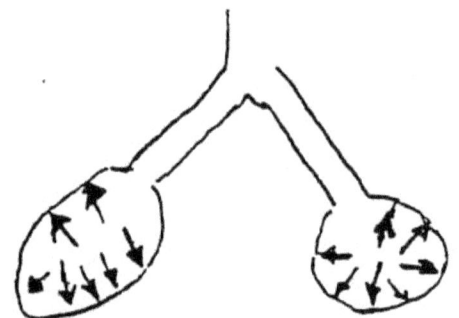

-10-

Continuing to look at the picture of me,
my bicycle pump and a balloon attached
to it:

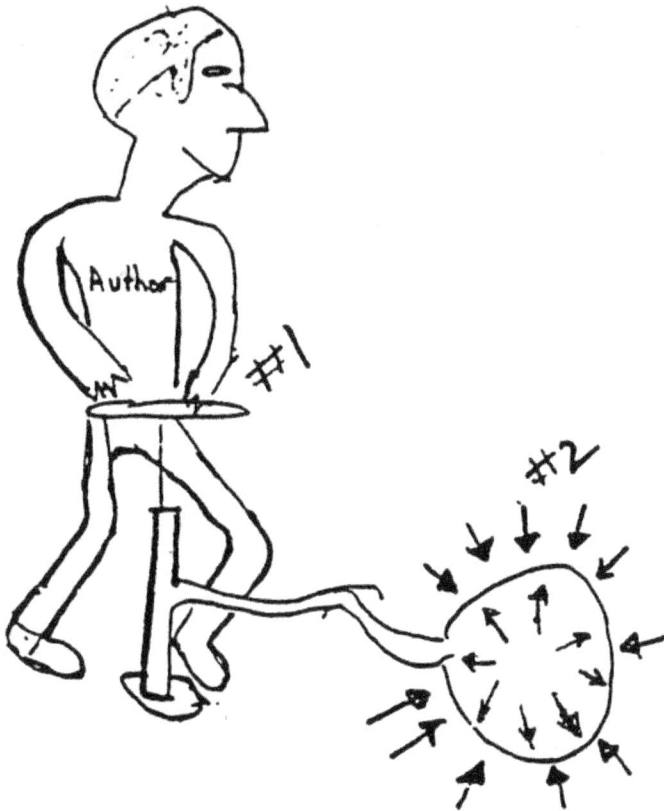

There are two pressures
here. #1 the downward
force   of the pump
piston on the air in the
pump and balloon and #2
the pressure of the
balloon that would like
to be in its normal
unexpended state.

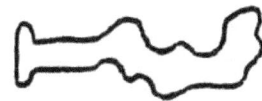

A molecule of air will go in the direction
of whatever pressure is greatest. We'll
call that difference in pressure the
pressure difference (makes sense). If we
look at an oxygen molecule in the hose

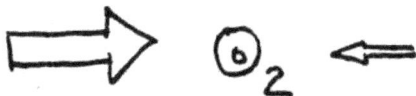

It will go in the direction of the greatest
pressure.

Or if the guy in the picture (me) let go
of the handle and squeezed the balloon,
the gas pressure within the balloon would
be transferred to an upward pressure on
the handle. The air molecules are traveling
in the direction of most pressure.

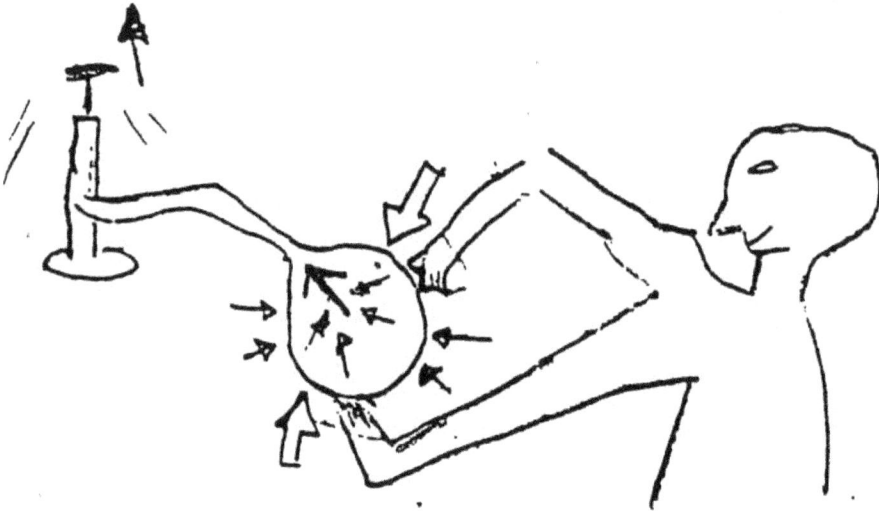

This is similar to our lungs breathing
out air by contracting and forcing out
the air by a pressure difference.

Diffusion

Diffusion is molecules getting through very small holes.

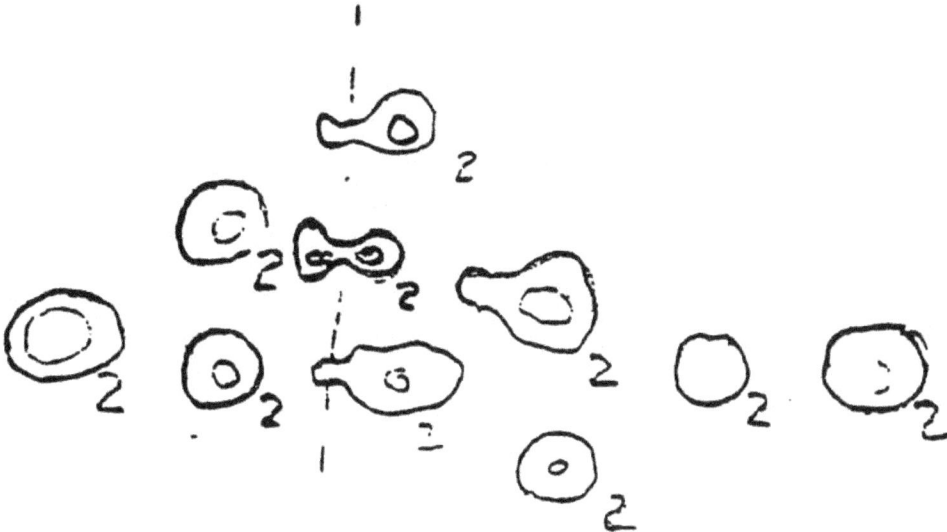

Here we see oxygen molecules slipping through small holes. This is very important because that is exactly what our lungs are - a very thin membrane with lots of very tiny holes.

If you spread out our lungs the whole surface area would be about the size of a tennis court (no kidding). The lungs allow O_2 through one way and CO_2 (carbon dioxide) the other way.

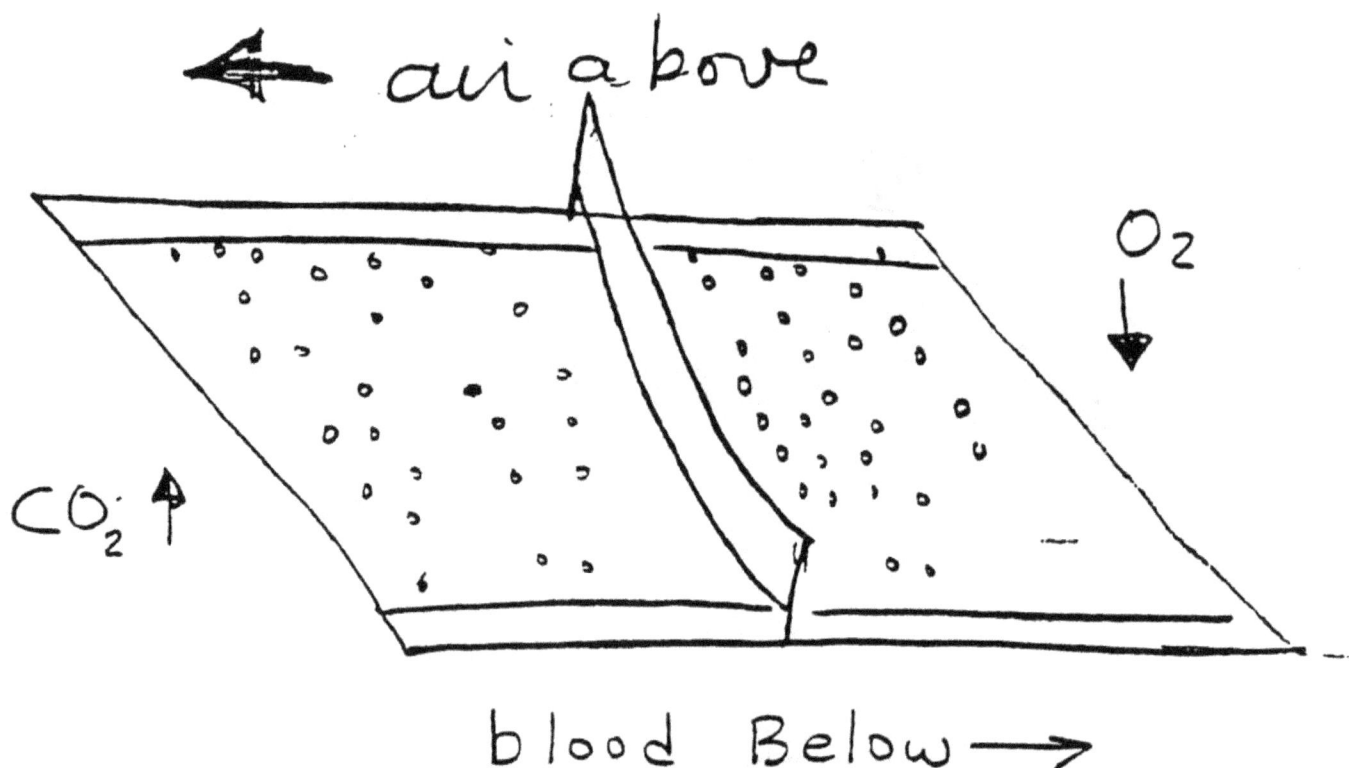

Air fills millions of tiny air sacks called alveoli. From there it crosses into the blood. The difference in pressure pushes them through tiny holes.

Diffusion

Generally gases (like air) respond to pressure. More pressure - more air transported through the small holes.

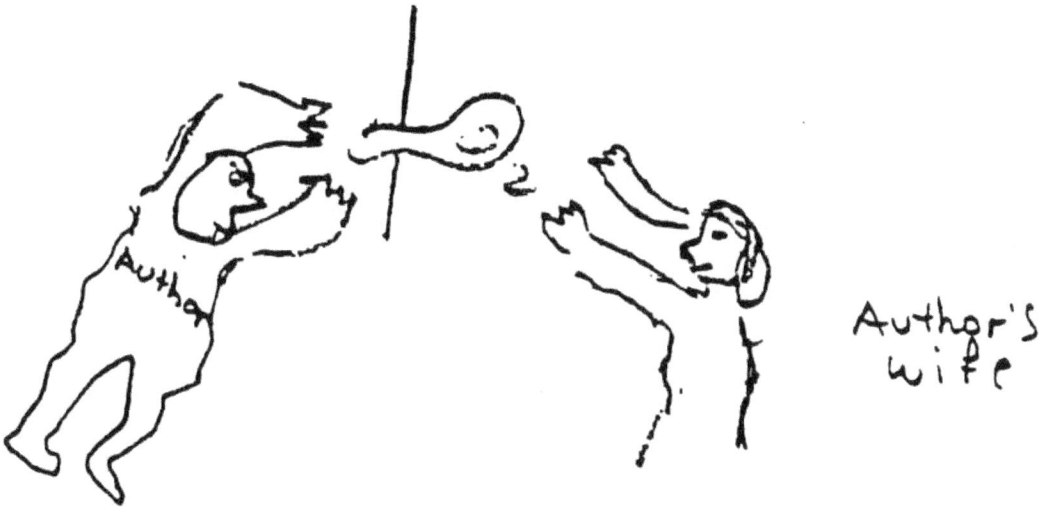

Author

Author's wife

Here the pressure difference will determine which way the oxygen goes.

For instance, when you kiss, the air will go from the mouth of the person breathing hardest.

Partial Pressure

When there is more than one gas, like O_2 and N_2 the total pressure is made up of the PARTIAL PRESSURES of each individual gas. If oxygen is 20% of the volume and nitrogen is 80%, the oxygen exerts 20% of the pressure and the nitrogen exerts 80% of the pressure.

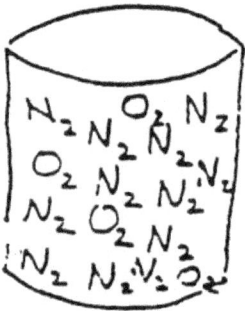

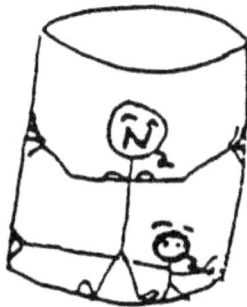

N_2 is exerting 4 times as much pressure as O_2.

Partial Pressure

If that can had millions of tiny holes
the nitrogen (N_2) would be pushed out by
the partial pressure of the nitrogen and
the oxygen would be pushed out by its
own partial pressure. You'll remember
that the nitrogen exerts four times as
much pressure.

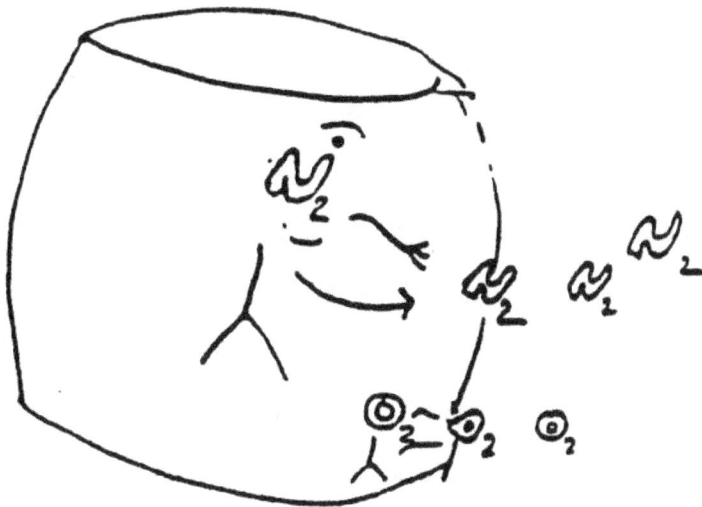

Partial Pressure

The important point here is that each gas acts under its own partial pressure - not the total pressure. In particular each gas diffuses through the lung based on its own partial pressure.

To be a little more accurate, you have to look at the partial pressure difference on either side of the lung - the blood side and the atmosphere side.

Lets look at a make believe example.

Partial Pressure
(Make Believe Example)

We have two chambers
separated by a
thin membrane - like our lungs:

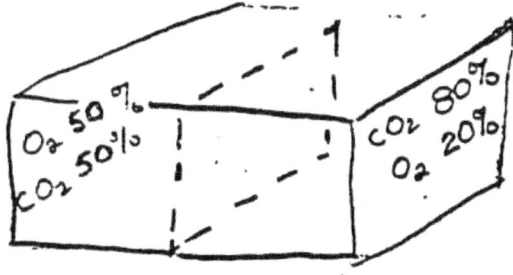

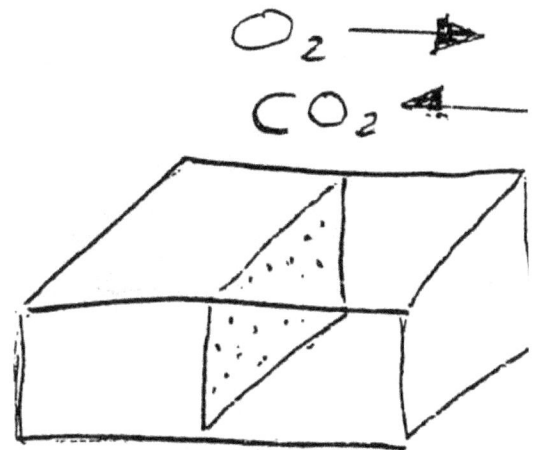

On one side there is 50% O_2 and 50% CO_2.
On the other side there is 80% CO_2 and
20% O_2. If the total pressure is the
same on both sides, the partial pressure
difference would cause the shift shown.
O_2 would cross the membrane in the
direction shown: 50% to 20% greater to
lesser pressure. CO_2 would travel and
cross the membrane in the opposite
direction, 80% to 20%.

As far as carbon dioxide is concerned, the oxygen isn't even there. The CO_2 is responding only to the pressure difference, The pressure is higher on the side where it is 80% of the volume. Remember: pressure of a gas is the force with which it attempts to move from one place to another at lower pressure.

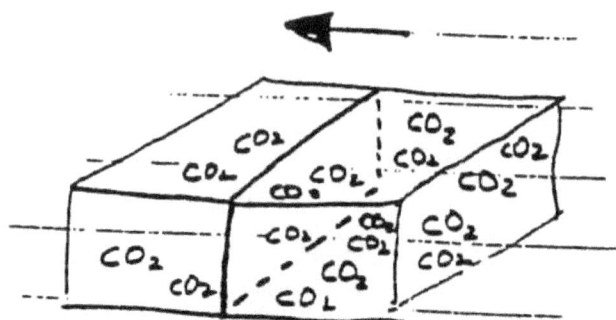

Similarly, the O_2 will travel in the direction of greater to less partial pressure.

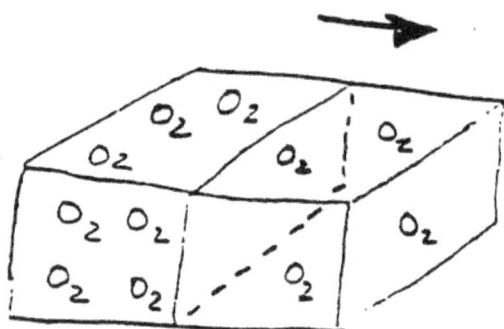

The individual gases will move through the membrane even though the **total** (not the partial) pressure is the same. They respond to their individual partial pressure difference.

GASES in LIQUIDS

Now we're going to look at how gases behave when they are dissolved in a liquid.

The reason is simple. That's exactly what blood is. For our purposes - to learn arterial blood gases - blood is water with some dissolved gases.

Let's look at "Fizzy Soda" which has CO_2 in water.

These are the bubbles in soda. The "fizz" tickles your nose.

Flat soda means No Fizz.

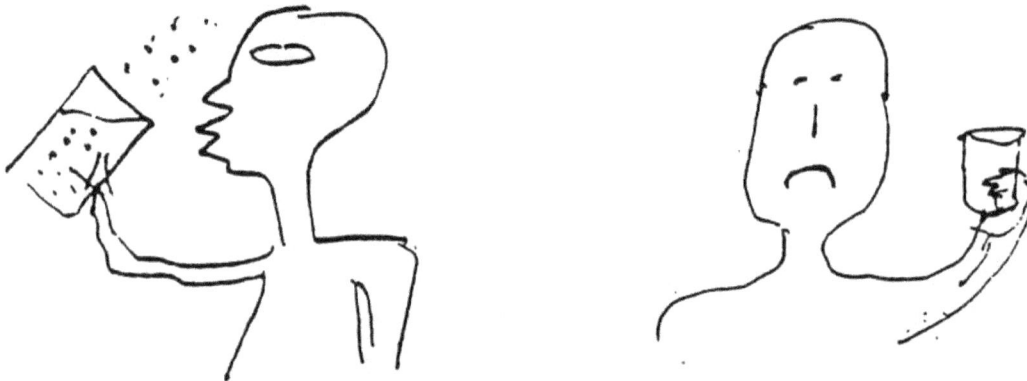

At the soda bottling plant

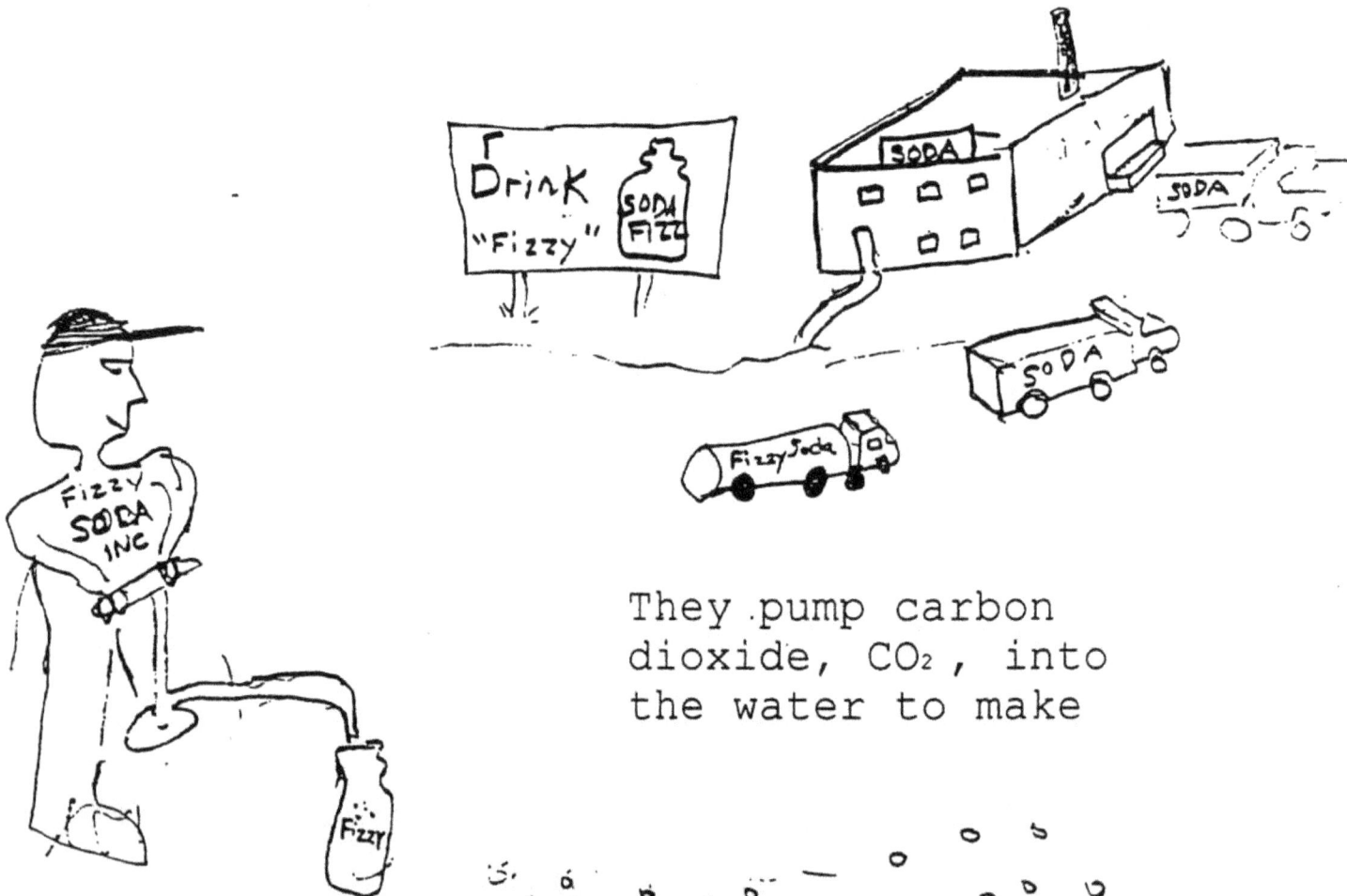

Drink "Fizzy"
SODA FIZZ
SODA
SODA
Fizzy Soda
SODA

They pump carbon dioxide, CO_2, into the water to make

Fizzy Soda Inc
Fizzy

Carbonated water

The amount of CO_2 depends
on the pressure. More
pressure means more CO_2
will go in.

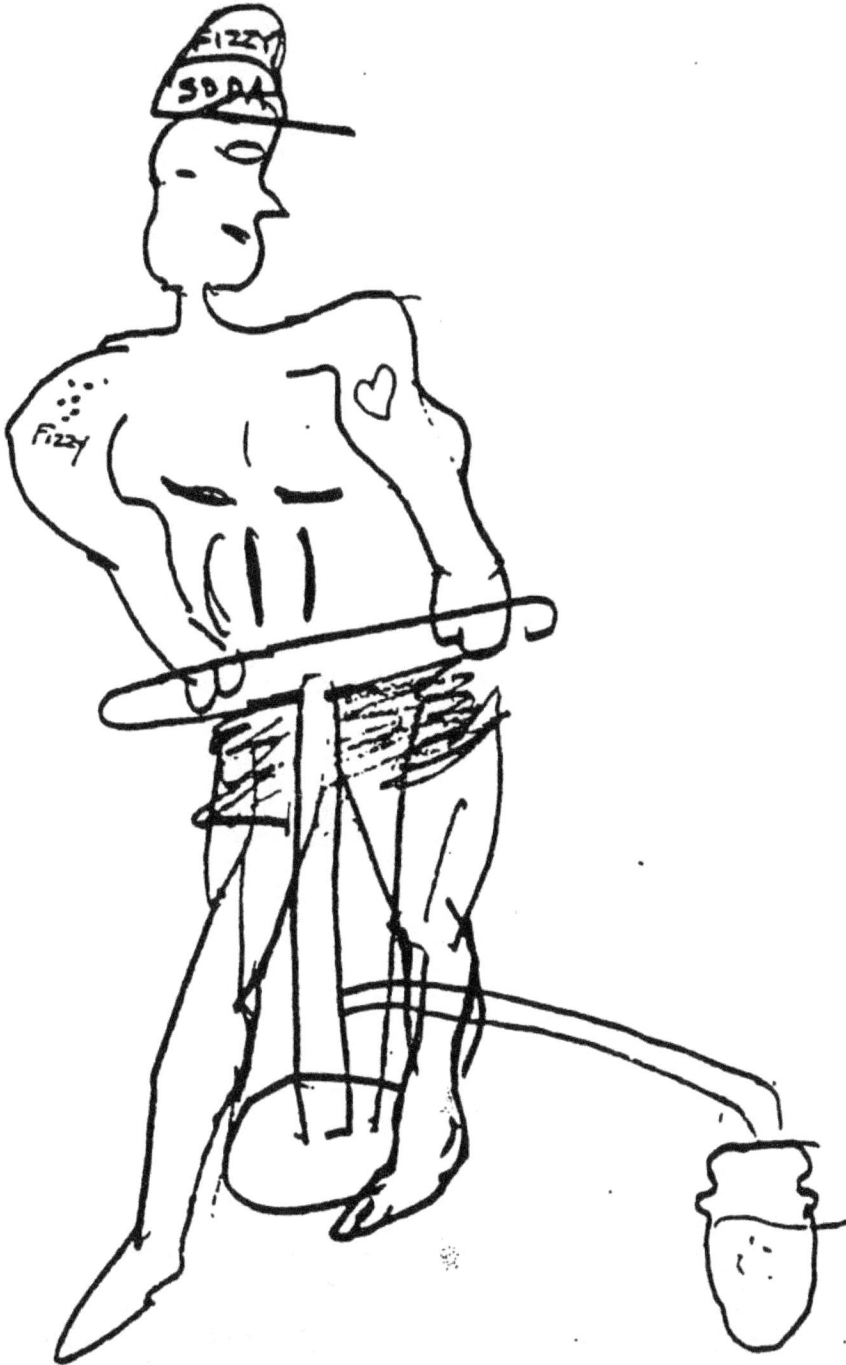

If the pressure of the gas (in this case CO_2) is greater inside the container than outside, it will fly out.

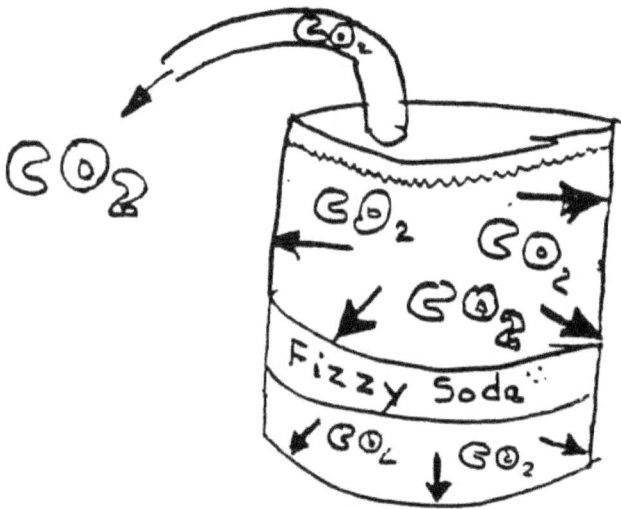

Keep in mind that we are working our way toward blood CO_2 and oxygen.

If the pressure of CO_2 is greater outside the fizzy soda can the CO_2 will flow inside. The extra pressure is supplied by the pump and me (my wife is "Sandy")

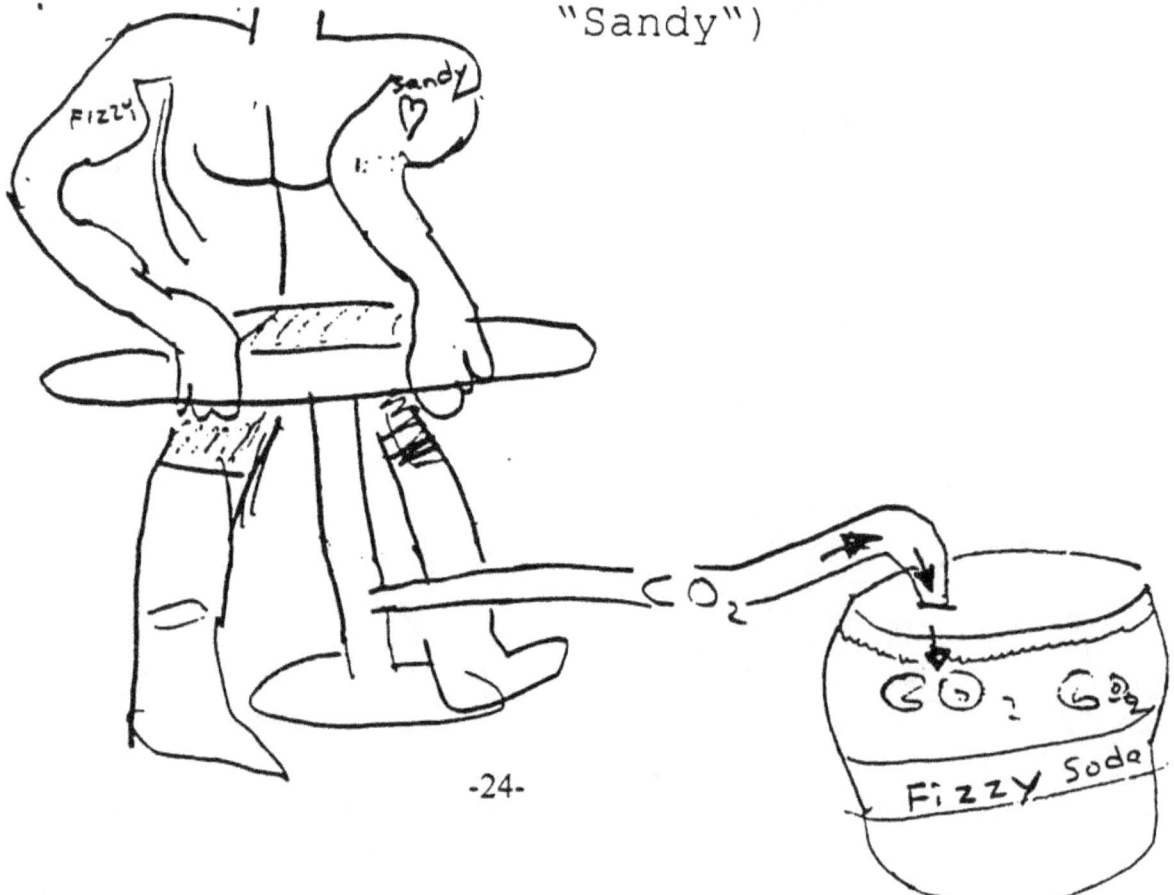

GASES and LIQUIDS

Both gases **and** liquids are composed of molecules like our friends O_2, N_2, H_2O.

Although most liquids look pretty dense, actually very large distances separate the molecules. The only difference between water

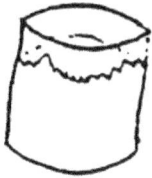

in this pan

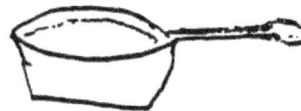

and water vapor or steam is the distance between the molecules.

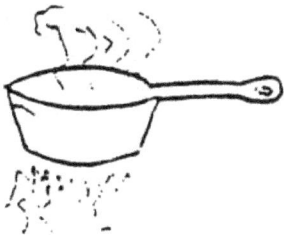

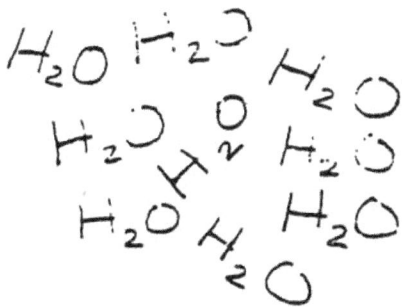

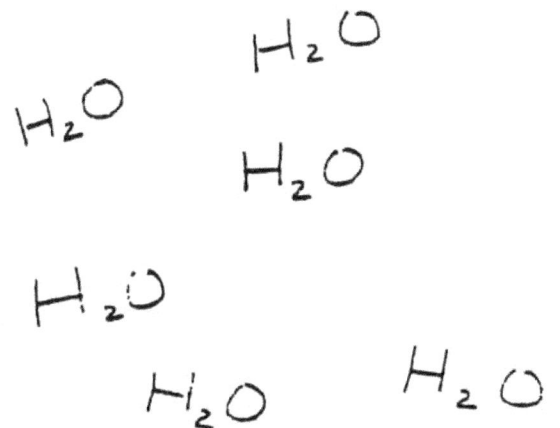

H_2O H_2O H_2O
H_2O H_2O H_2O
H_2O H_2O H_2O

H_2O H_2O
H_2O H_2O
H_2O
H_2O H_2O

What does DISSOLVED Mean?

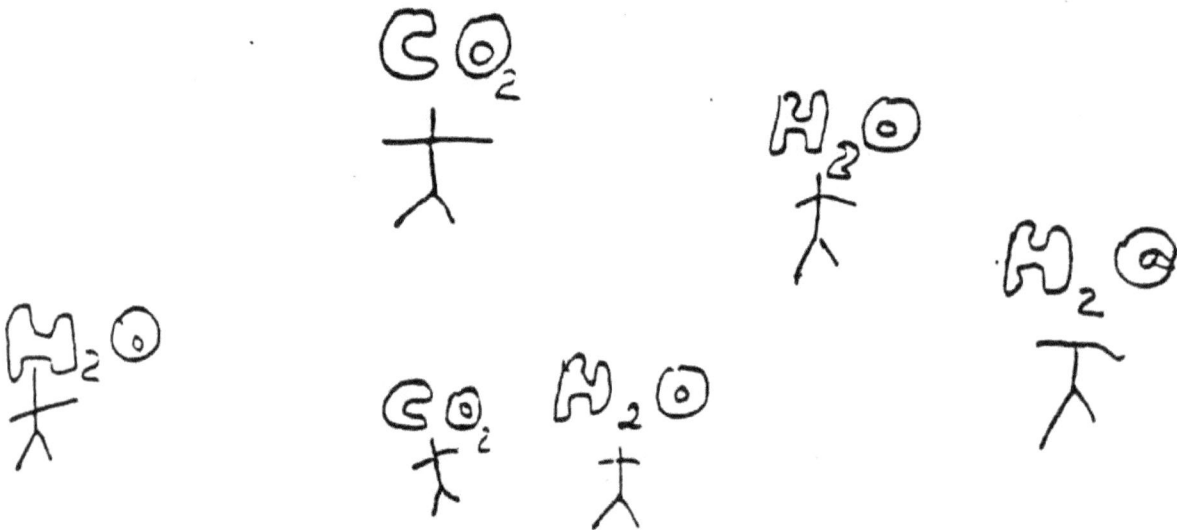

When two different kinds of molecules mix and one of them is a gas (like carbon dioxide) and the other a liquid (like water) its called dissolved.

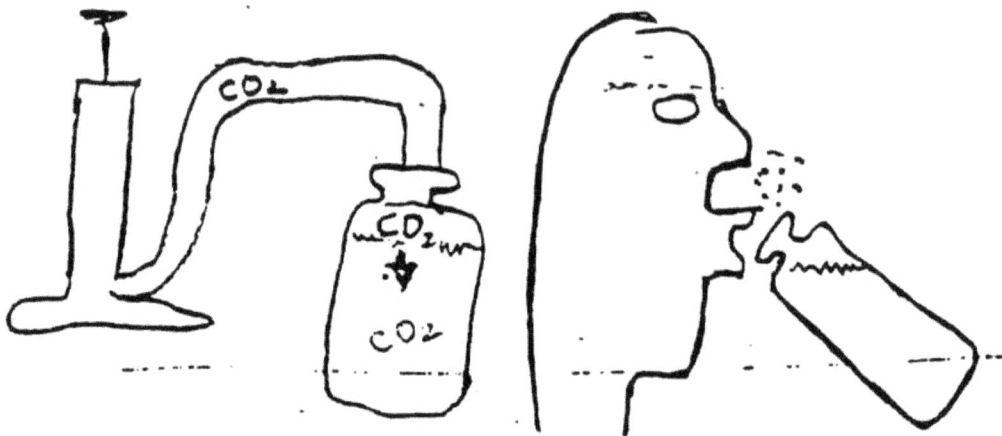

To see how quickly they separate just shake your soda before you drink it.

The important point here is that the gas pressure only depends on how much of the gas is in the container. It is unaffected by the liquid.

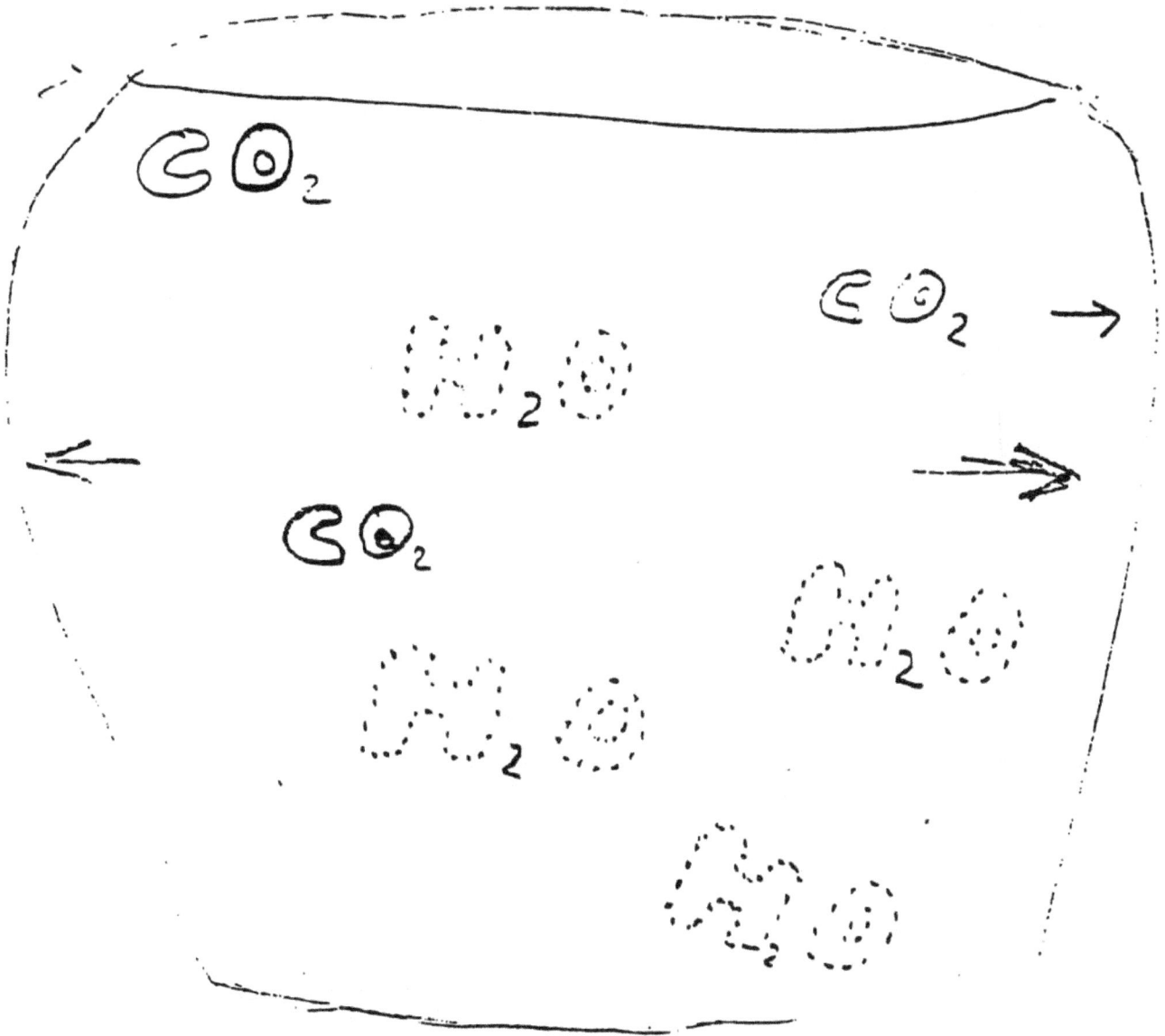

As far as the dissolved gas is concerned the water isn't even there at all. Very self centered.

TWO Gases Dissolved in Water

If oxygen is also dissolved in the carbonated water we have two gases dissolved in the water.

The important point is that the CO_2 is totally unaffected by the O_2.

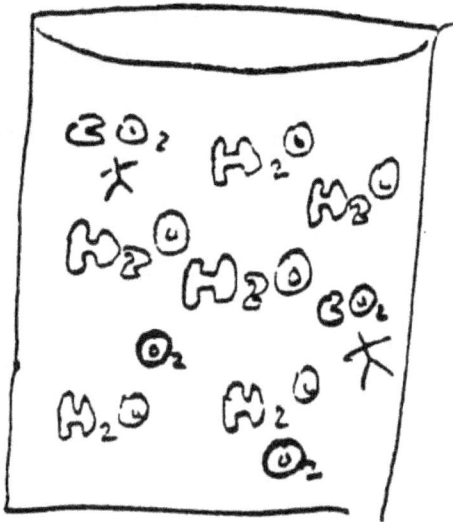

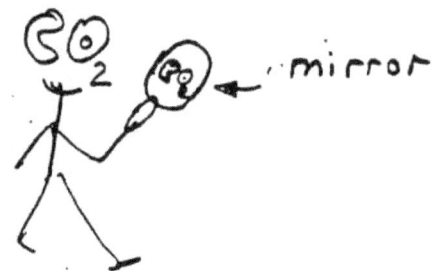

He is totally self centered

But that's O.K. The O_2 doesn't care about any other gas in the same can. As far as O_2 is concerned, it is the only gas in the can.

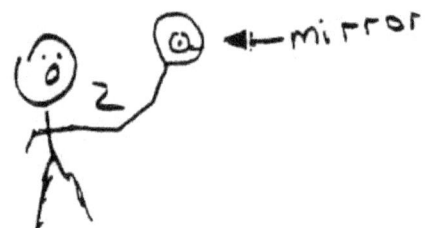

Two Gases

I think (hope) we understand that two gases mixed together don't care about each other.

And the same is true of more than one gas dissolved in a liquid (like our blood).

Throughout this book we'll see how oxygen and carbon dioxide behave dissolved in our blood.

That lengthy explanation of two gases dissolved in one liquid is OUR OWN BLOOD. The two gases are carbon dioxide (CO_2) and oxygen (O_2).

Lets start with this pan made of very thin membranes with microscopic holes - not exactly cast iron.

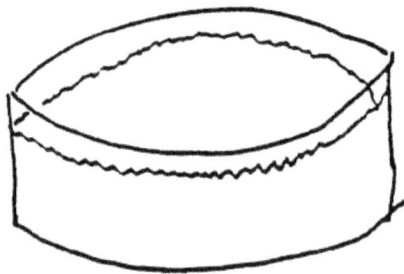

Oxygen is "pumped" (diffuses) into the
blood through the lungs by higher pressure
in the atmosphere. Partial pressure of
O_2 is 100mm Hg in the lung and 37mm Hg in
the blood.

LUNG 100

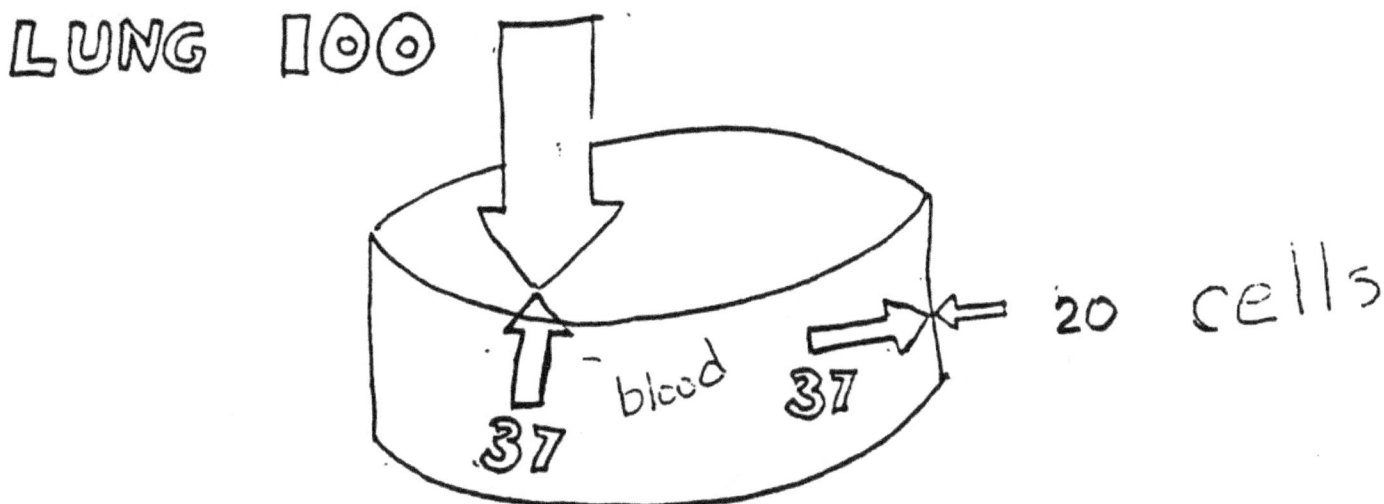

From the capillaries, oxygen diffuses into
every cell in our body. The pressure
difference causes this. Partial pressure
of oxygen in the cells varies from 20mm Hg
to 35mm Hg.

At the same time, the same blood is transporting carbon dioxide from the cells. We'll see how the cells produce carbon dioxide in about 6 pages. Can you wait?

Carbon dioxide partial pressure in the

0.3 (lungs)

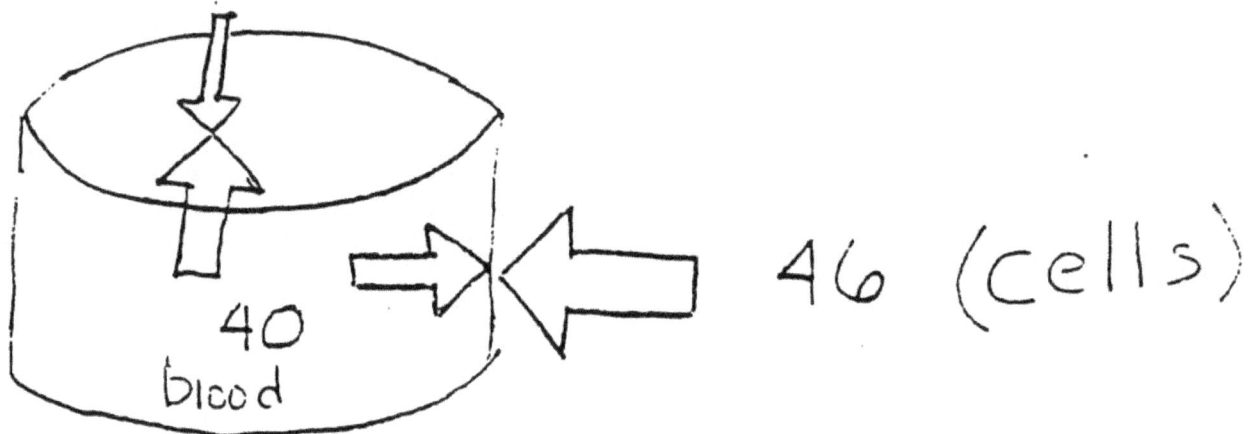

40
blood

46 (cells)

tissues is greater than 46mm Hg. P_{CO_2} partial pressure of CO_2) in the blood is 40. Actually we'll see the range is 35 to 45mm Hg. Since its lower in the blood than in the cells, CO_2 partial pressure in the atmosphere is 0.3mm Hg.

The Cast in Blood Gases

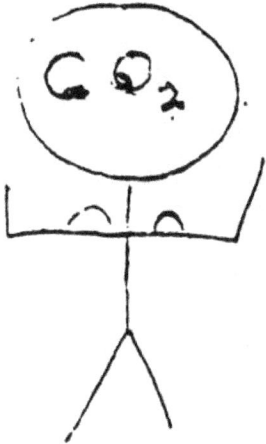

Here is the partial pressure
of carbon dioxide. Notice
his biceps.

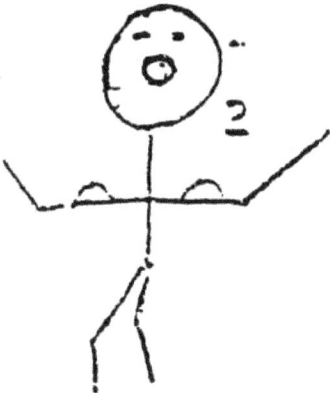

Here is the partial pressure
of oxygen. Look for the
chemical symbol and the
biceps.

Now that you understand Partial Pressure,
let's look at...

Oxygen Saturation
"O_2 Sat"   "Sat"

There is a lot of confusion about the
difference between Oxygen Saturation (SaO_2)
and Partial Pressure of Oxygen (PaO_2).

The most noticeable is that an oxygen saturation
is obtained by a pulse oxymeter and oxygen partial
pressure is obtained by arterial blood gas (ouch!).

We will review.

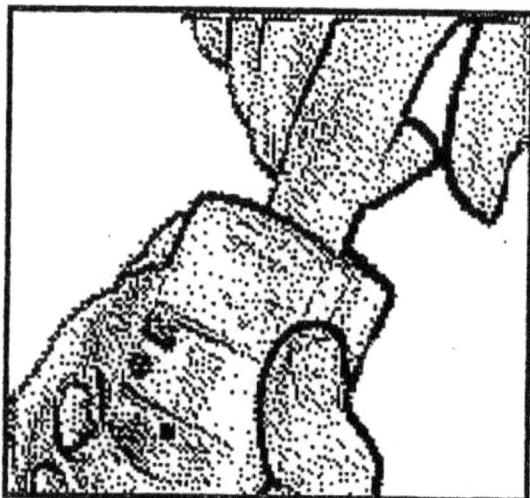

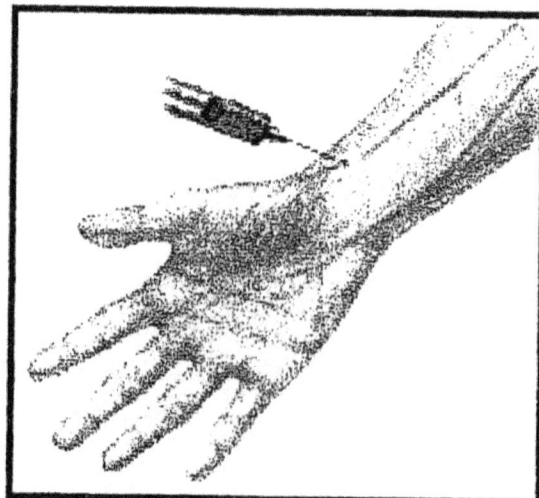

Pressure gradient...
think, "flows downhill."

There is a big oxygen (PaO_2) pressure difference (104 vs. 40) between alveola air in the lungs and pulmonary veinous blood which is returning to the lungs.

The oxygen pressure is much higher in alveolas (104mmHg) than it is in the blood returning to the lungs (40mmHg.

This pressure gradient pushes the oxygen through the alveolas into the blood.

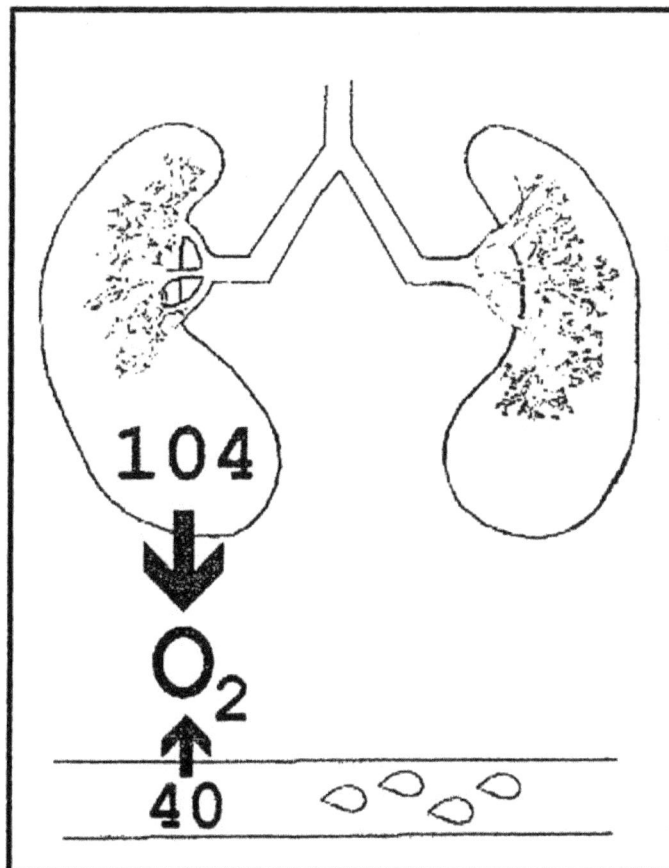

Far away from your heart in say, your index finger the opposite happens. The blood gets to the capillaries pretty much the same way it left the heart with a PaO_2 of about 97. That is because there is no exchange of oxygen until the blood reaches the capillaries. That's because there are no holes for the oxygen to sneak through.

The cells of your index finger have burned oxygen (from pointing). The partial pressure of oxygen in finger cells is about 30. Since 97mmHg is higher than 30mmHg, oxygen flows from the blood into the cells. Along the way, the blood looses oxygen to the point where the PaO_2 is 40 by the time it gets to the veins and then returns to the heart.

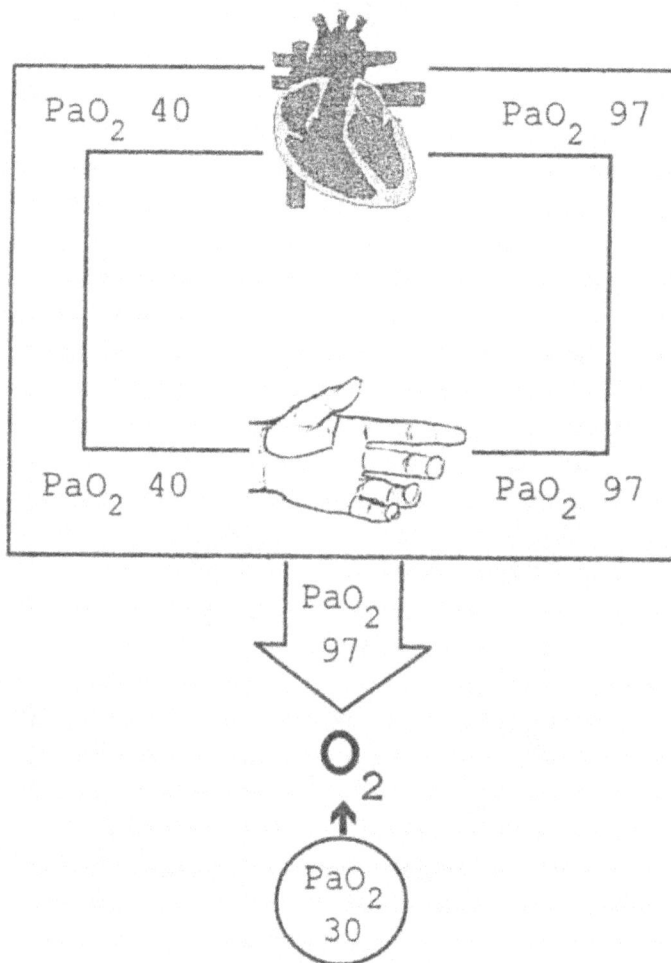

Pressure gradient...
think, "flows downhill."

The pressure gradient pushes oxygen through tiny holes.
This is called diffusion.

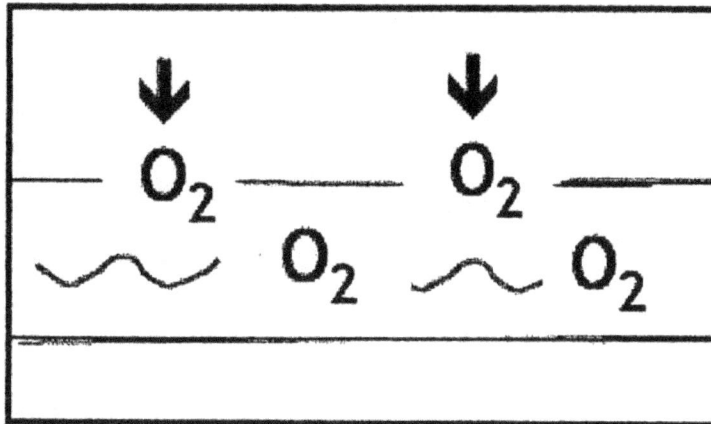

Red Blood Cells
& Hemoglobin

In the blood, red blood cells (RBC) carry oxygen to the six trillion cells in the body.

We are going to see the red blood cell (RBC) as a pickup truck. The cargo area is hemoglobin, because each oxygen attaches to the hemoglobin part of the red blood cell.

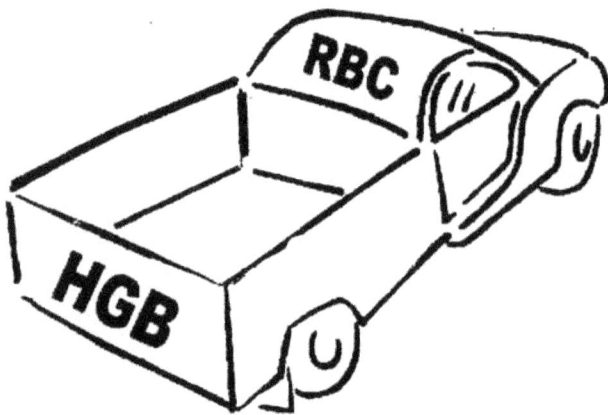

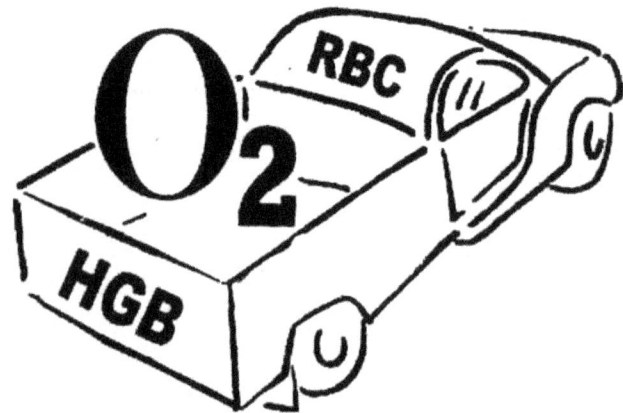

Red Blood Cells
& Hemoglobin

After the oxygen diffuses into the blood, 98% of it attaches to the hemoglobin on each red blood cell.

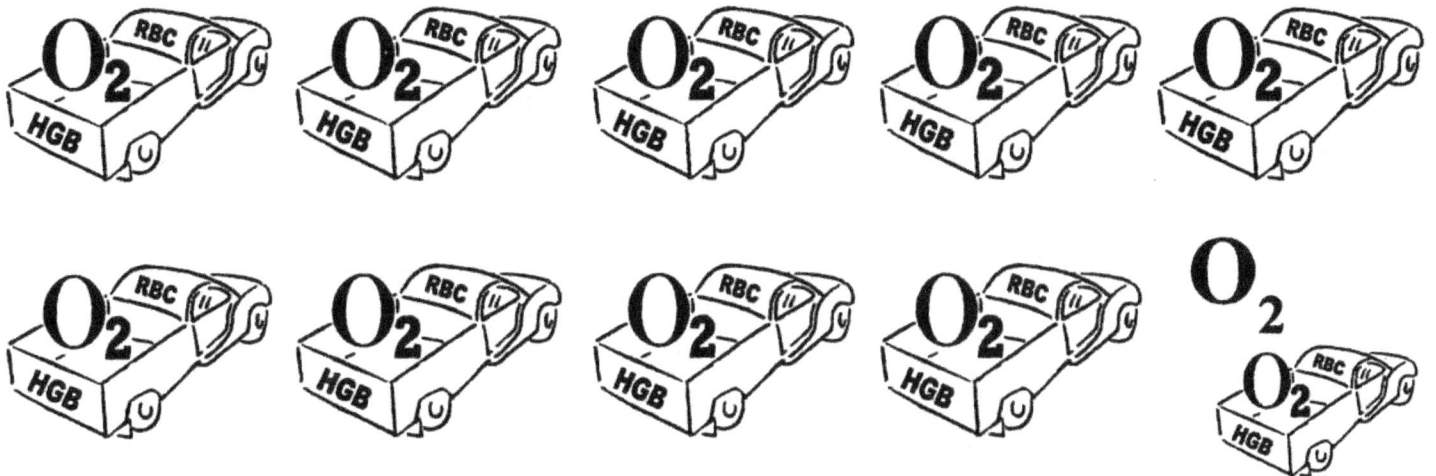

A very small amount, about 2% floats freely in the bloodstream.

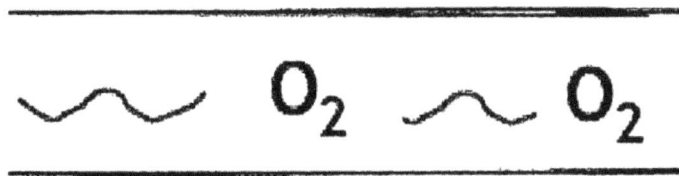

Definition:
Partial Pressure of Oxygen

The partial pressure of oxygen (PaO_2) is obtained from an ABG stick (ouch!). It is a measurement of the oxygen pressure of the oxygen floating freely in the blood (not attached to hemoglobin).

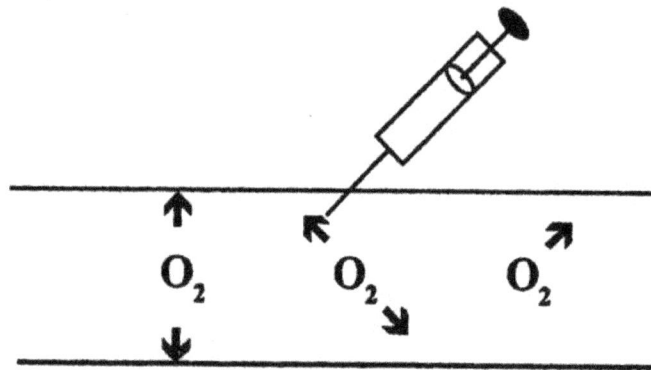

Definition:
Oxygen Saturation

Oxygen Saturation is the percentage
of red blood cells (hemoglobin) that have
an oxygen molecule attached to it.

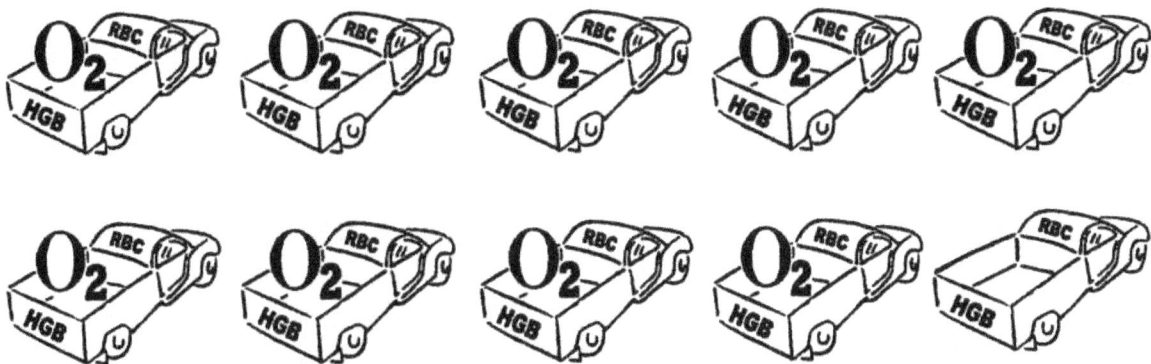

This is 90% saturation. Note that one in ten
does not have an oxygen attached.

Relationship between Oxygen Pressure (PaO$_2$) and Oxygen Saturation (SaO$_2$)

The amount of oxygen that attaches to the hemoglobin (O$_2$ Saturation) depends on the partial pressure (PaO$_2$) of the oxygen floating freely in the bloodstream.

Here we see a PaO$_2$ of 40mmHg pushes the oxygen to combine with 70% of the red blood cells.

More PaO$_2$ more SaO$_2$
Here we see a PaO$_2$ of 60 pushes the oxygen to combine with 90% of the red blood cells.

40 ↓
O$_2$

↓ 60
O$_2$

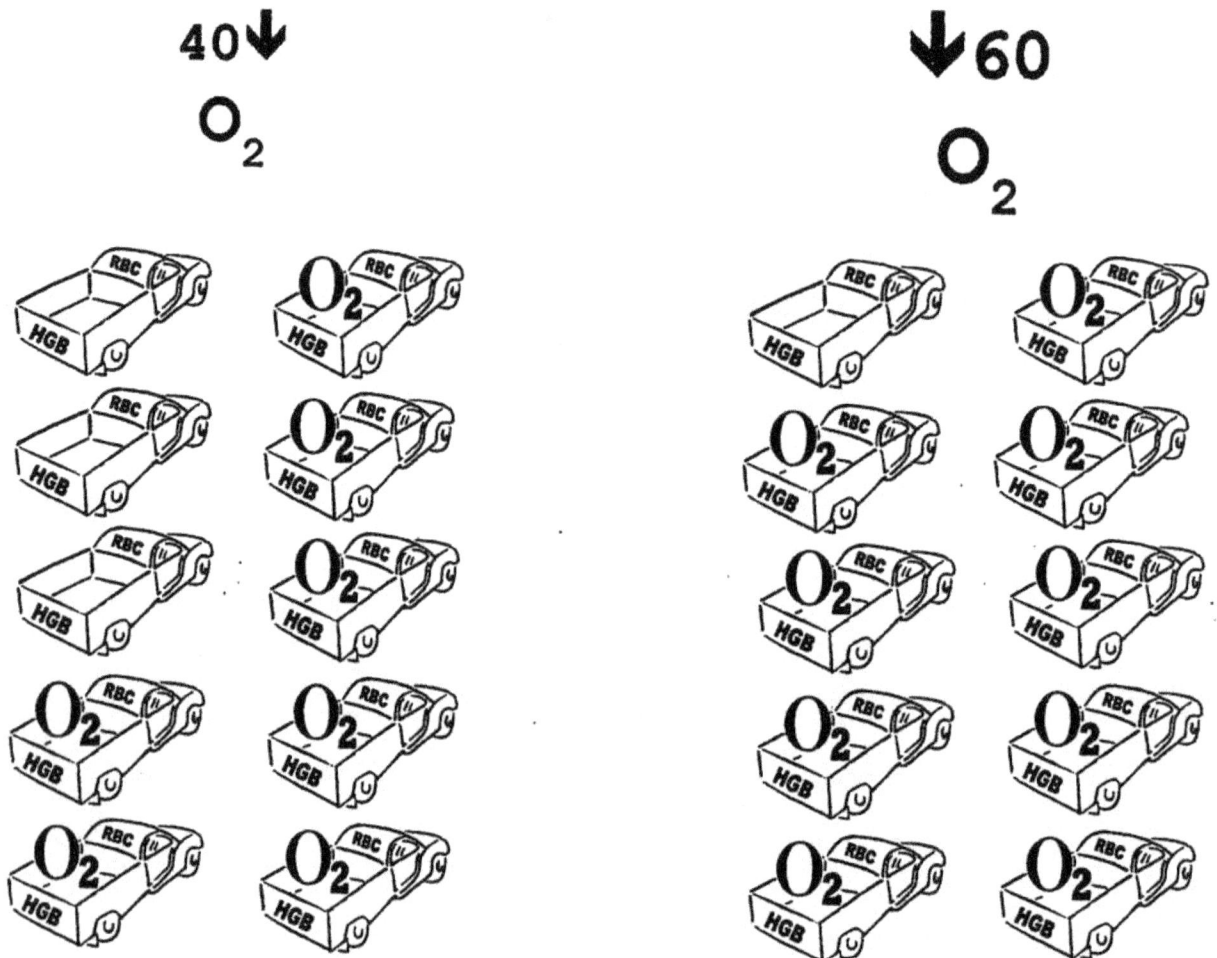

Here's one more example...

A PaO_2 of 100 (which is a normal number for oxygenated blood leaving the lungs) causes an oxygen to attach to 97% of the red blood cells. (97%O_2 sat).

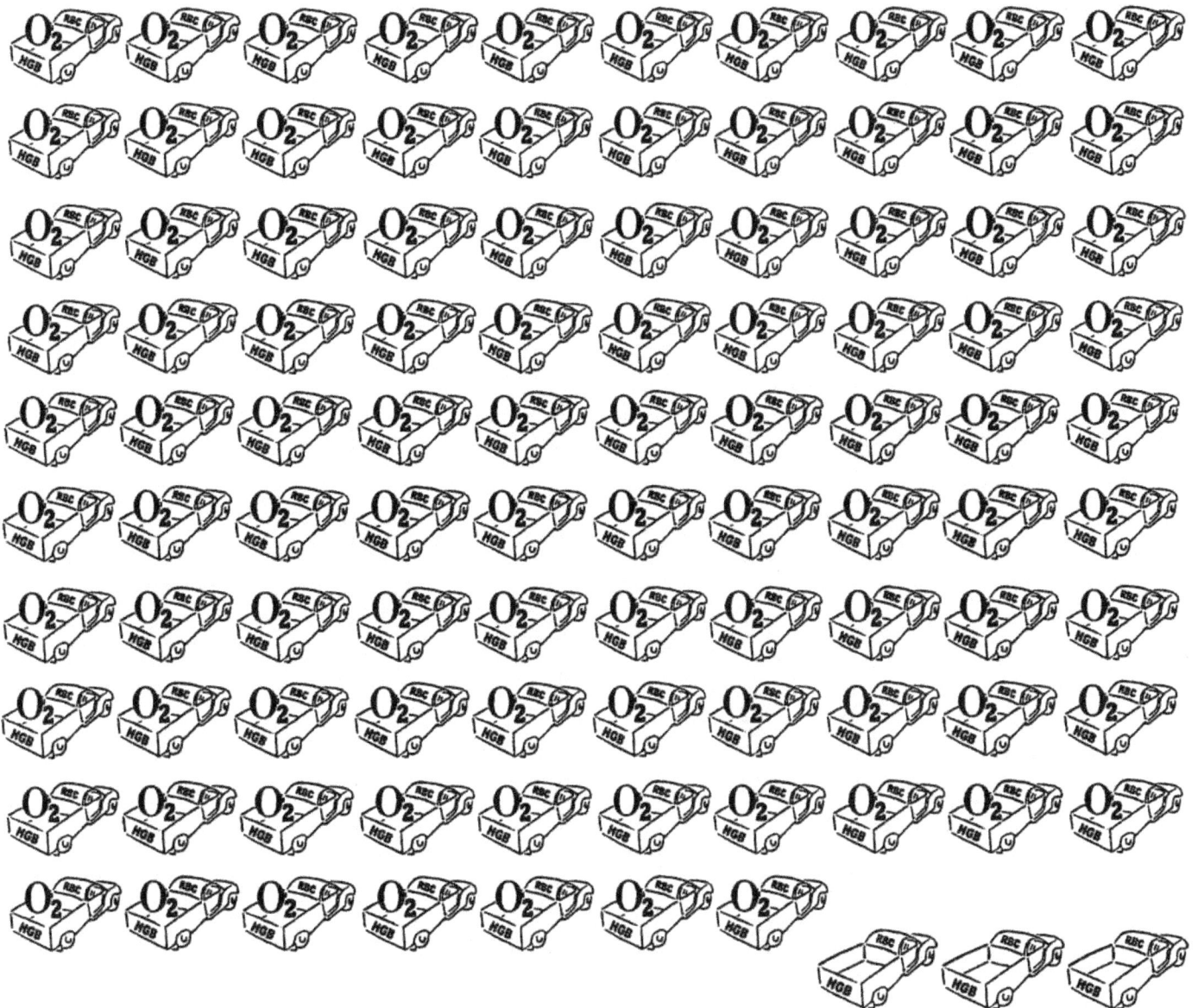

Oxygen Hemoglobin Dissociation Curve

The relationship between oxygen saturation and Partial Oxygen Pressure is shown on a graph called the Oxygen Hemoglobin Dissociation Curve.

Here is a graph of the three examples presented earlier:

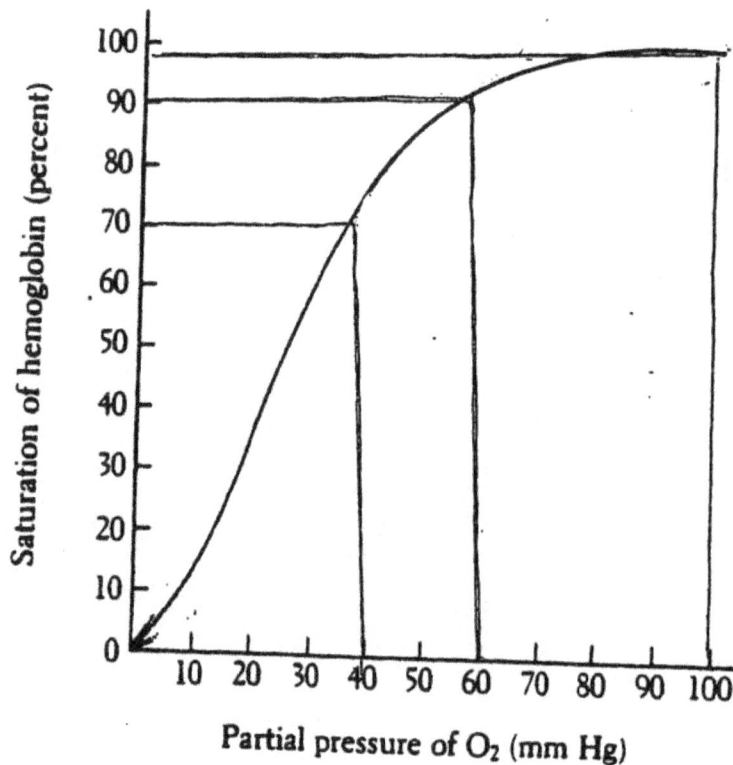

At this point in time...

You only need to know two things:

❶ High surrounding oxygen pressure (like 104 in the lungs) force oxygen into the blood. In the blood, high oxygen partial pressure (like 97mmHg in bright red freshly oxygenated blood) pushes oxygen to attach to hemoglobin and cause high oxygen saturations.

❷ Low surrounding oxygen partial pressures (like 30mmHg in the skin cells of your big toe) allow oxygen to diffuse from the blood where the partial pressure is higher. The oxygen flows from the hemoglobin to the plasma and then through the capillary to the skin cell.

All the Chemistry
You'll Need to Know
(honest)

Oxygen.   As a gas oxygen floats around in pairs.   That's why we write O_2.

Carbon.   Carbon is an element that enters our body in the form of food, mash potatoes and Snickers.   These long molecules get into the blood by way of the small intestines. From the blood it goes to the cells where sugar is "burned" to give us energy.   The cells break down sugars to carbon dioxide and water and liberate lots of energy.   The carbon dioxide and water return to blood which flows through the lungs where CO_2 is exhaled.

We eat carbon in the
form of sugar.

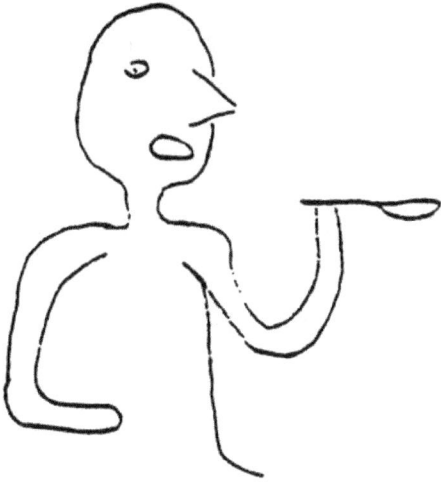

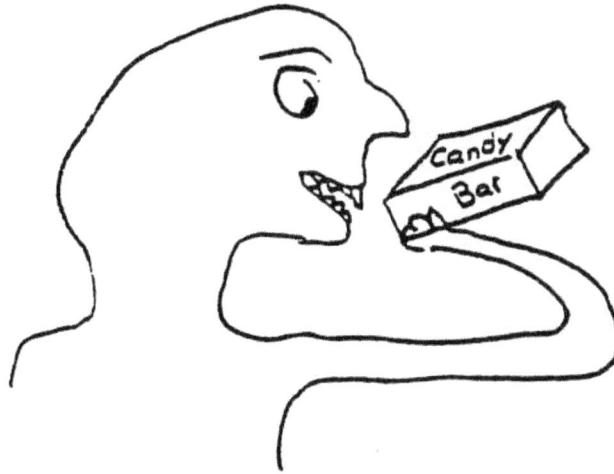

Which looks like this -
long strings of carbon
and oxygen.

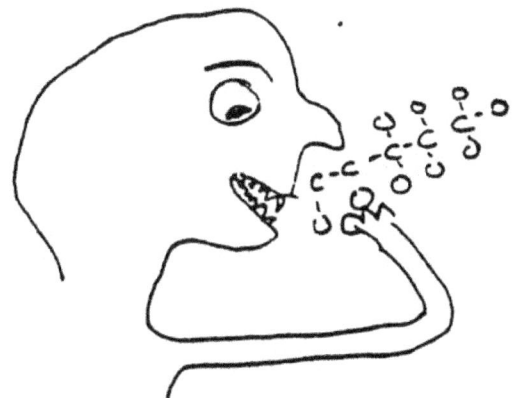

Metabolism

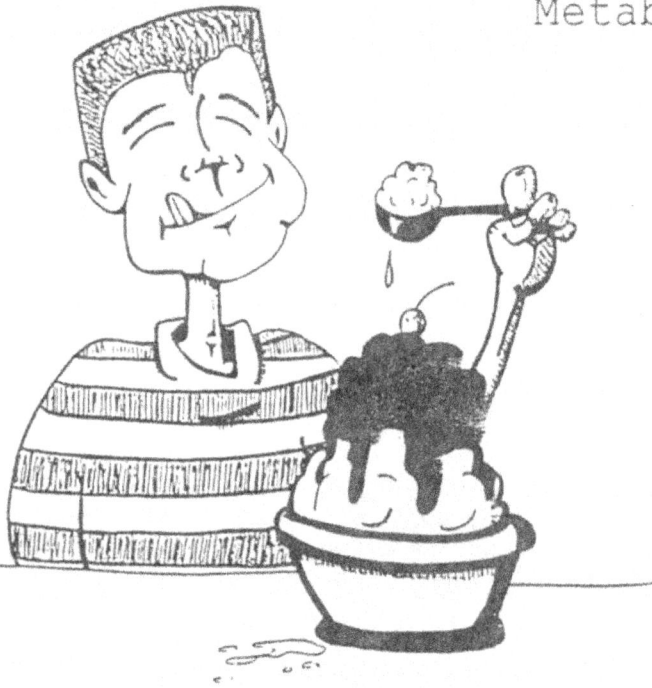

This is the first step in the metabolism of carbohydrates.

(1) Glucose, the Snickers bar and McDonald's french fries enter into the blood stream from the intestines.

(2) Oxygen enters your blood from the lungs.

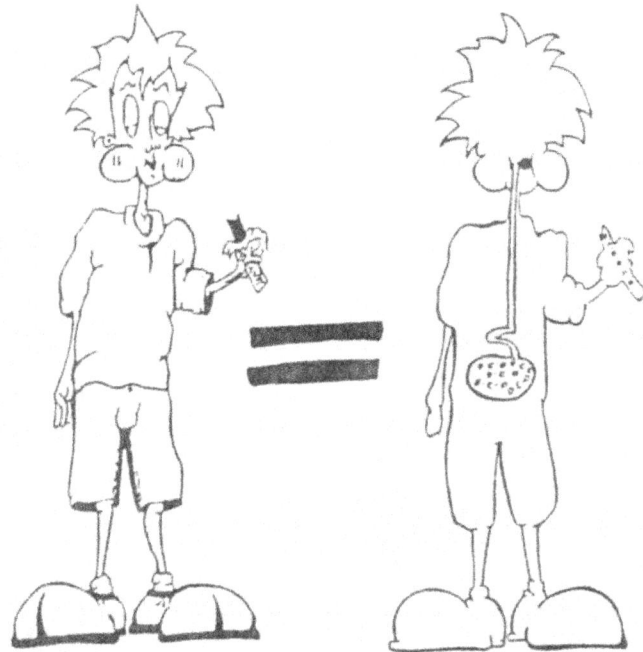

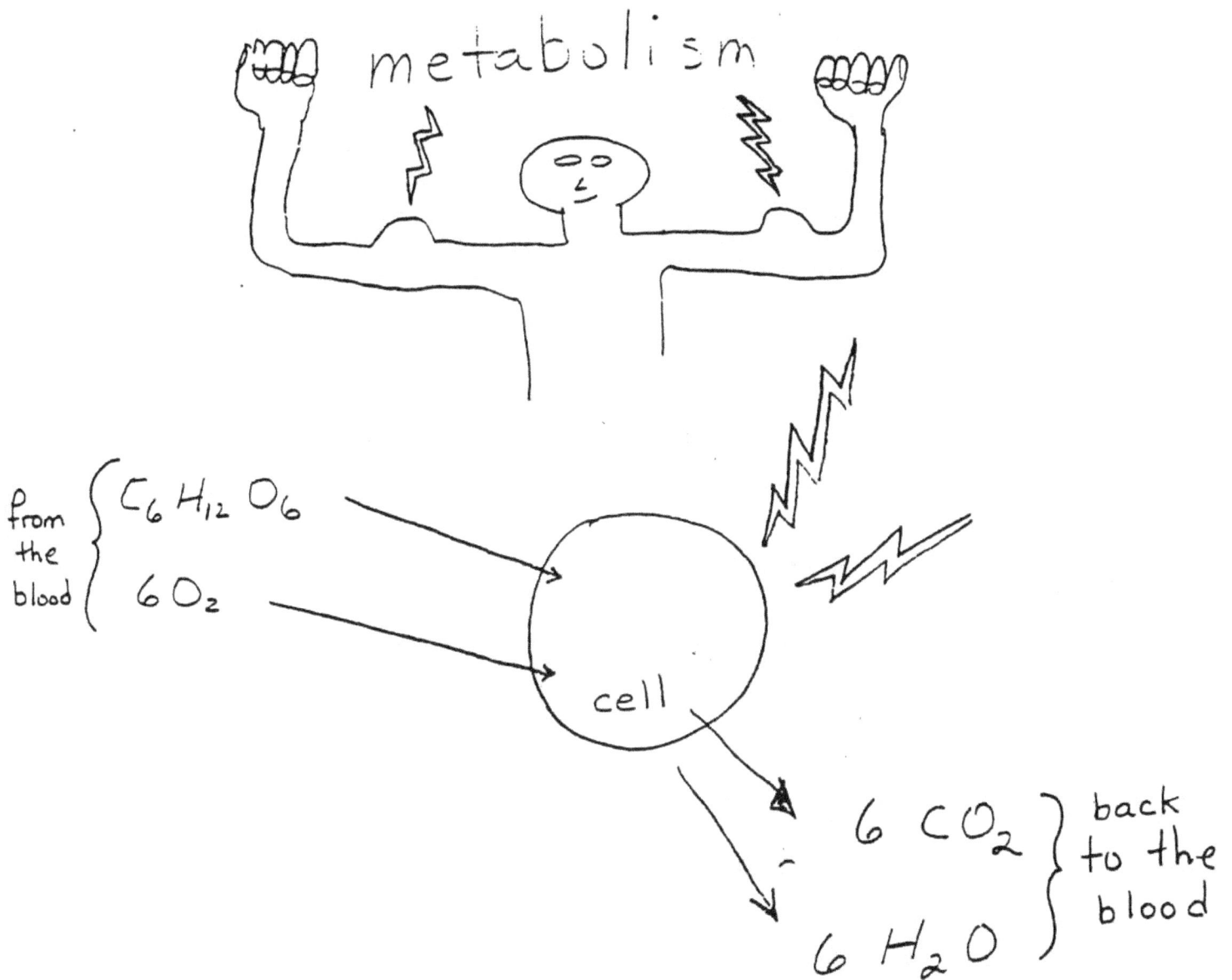

metabolism

from the blood { $C_6H_{12}O_6$

$6O_2$

cell

$6CO_2$ } back to the blood

$6H_2O$

From the blood, sugar and oxygen enter all the cells of your body (like in your brain to read this and in your fingers to turn the page). The sugar and oxygen reaction in the cells give off energy. The end products of this reaction go back to the blood.

pH

The correct number of hydrogen ions (H+) is very, very important to our well-being. In fact, slight deviations mean death. The hydrogen concentration in our blood is called "pH" (pee aych). The H in pH stands for Hydrogen. It would take forever to explain how the pH number reflects the concentration of H+ ions in the blood. Just remember three things:

#1: Normal pH values in our body are

7.35 to 7.45

#2: As pH value goes down it means more H+ floating around in our blood. When pH is less than 7.35 there are too many H+ ions and that's called Acidosis.

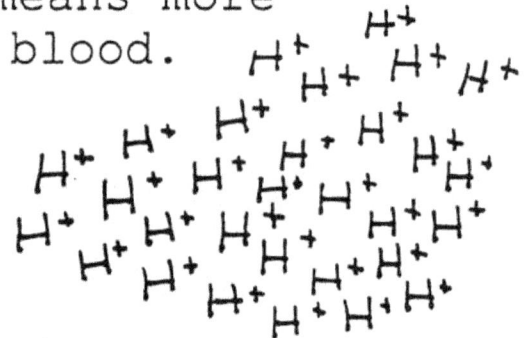

#3: When the pH goes up it means fewer H+ ions. That's called Alkalosis. pH values greater than 7.45 are Alkalotic.

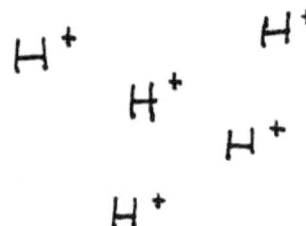

pH (continued)

I know you saw this explanation before. It's quite important and you'll see it again:

Our body gets its energy when all 6 trillion cells "burn" oxygen and sugar, H_2O and $C_6H_{10}O_5$. When oxygen and sugar react they form carbon dioxide and water.

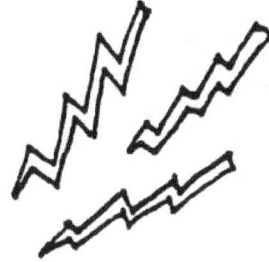

CO_2 and H_2O leave the cell and enter the blood stream. In the blood some CO_2 floats freely. And some H_2O and CO_2 joins to form carbonic acid (H_2CO_3).

Carbonic acid is a major source of H+ ions. A small percentage of carbonic acid throws off an H+ by breaking down into H+ and HCO_3-.

The first value in arterial blood gases will always be the concentration of H+ ions the pH.

pH (continued)

"Bicarb"

Blood gases also have the Bicarbonate level. We saw how carbonic acid can break down to bicarbonate and hydrogen ions.

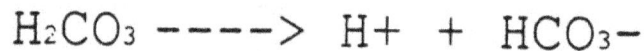

$$H_2CO_3 ----> H+ + HCO_3-$$

The opposite can also happen: bicarb can combine with H+ ions to form carbonic acid.

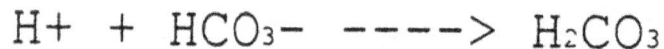

$$H+ + HCO_3- ----> H_2CO_3$$

That equation says that bicarb can "absorb" acid. A good example of that reaction would be baking soda, sodium bicarbonate absorbing excess acid in your stomach.

In the blood (which this book is all about),
if there is too much carbonic acid and too
many H+ ions, bicarbonate can come to the
rescue.   Lots of bicarbonate ions HCO_3 can
grab the H+ ions and take them out of
circulation.

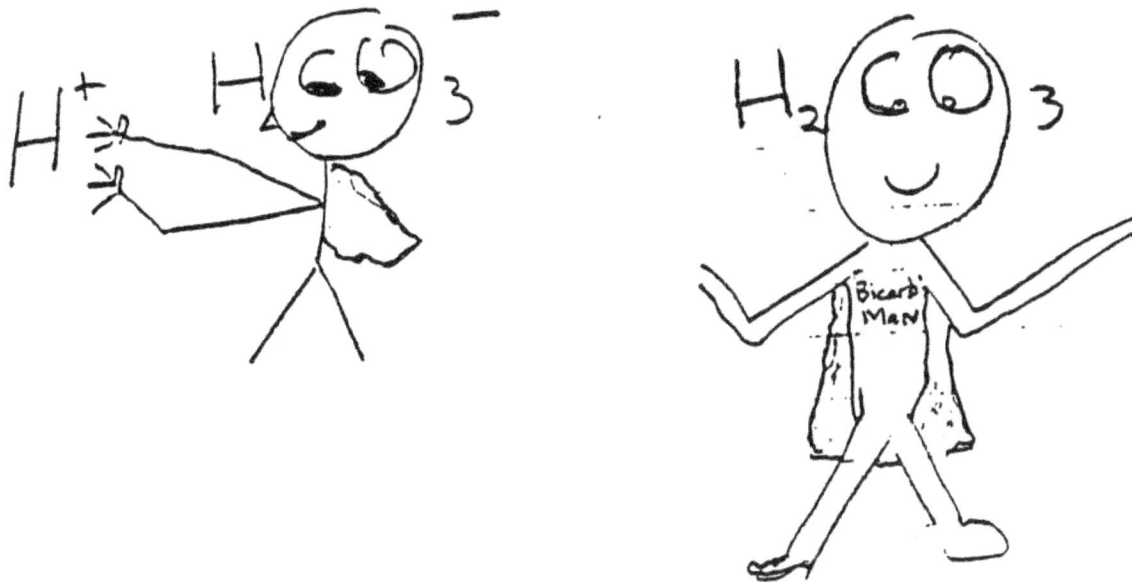

Or the opposite can happen.   If there are
too many bicarb ions floating around

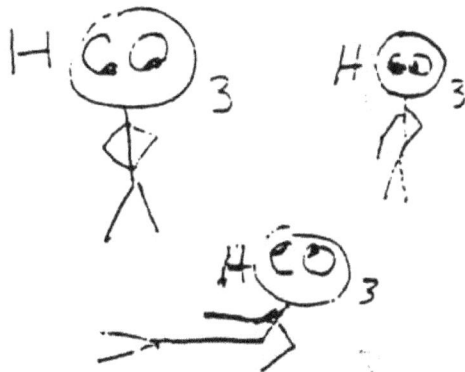

A bunch of H+ ions could round 'em up and
turn 'em into carbonic acid.

WHY BREATH?

Reason #1

OXYGEN

All 6,000,000,000,000 cells in your body
need oxygen.

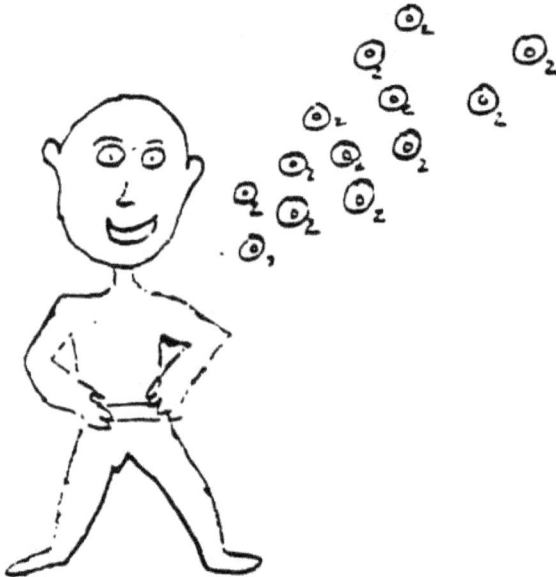

(more on this to follow)

"Respiration is oxygen going into the
blood and carbon dioxide getting out
of the blood."

WHY BREATH?

Reason #2

CO_2

Breathing gets rid of carbon dioxide
which all 6,000,000,000,000 cells in
your body need to get rid of

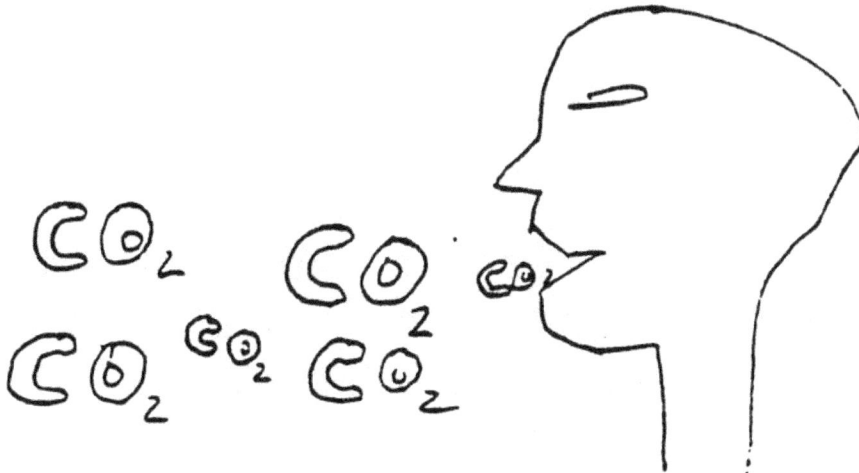

CO_2 CO_2 CO_2
CO_2 CO_2 CO_2

"Breathing is oxygen going into the
   blood and carbon dioxide getting out
   of the blood."

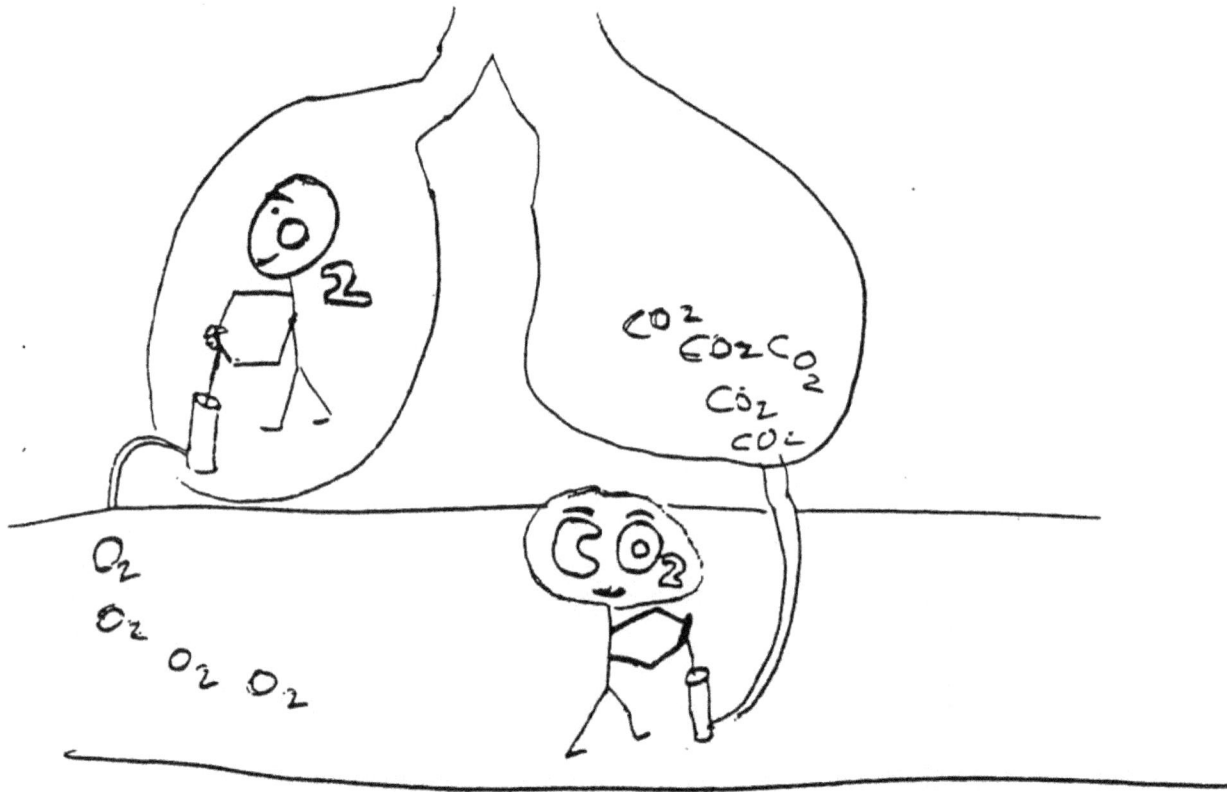

The exchange of gases in the lungs takes place between alveolar air and venous blood traveling through very small capillaries O_2 diffuses down the "ol' pressure gradient." It goes from greater pressure to lower pressure. CO_2 does the same thing in the opposite direction.

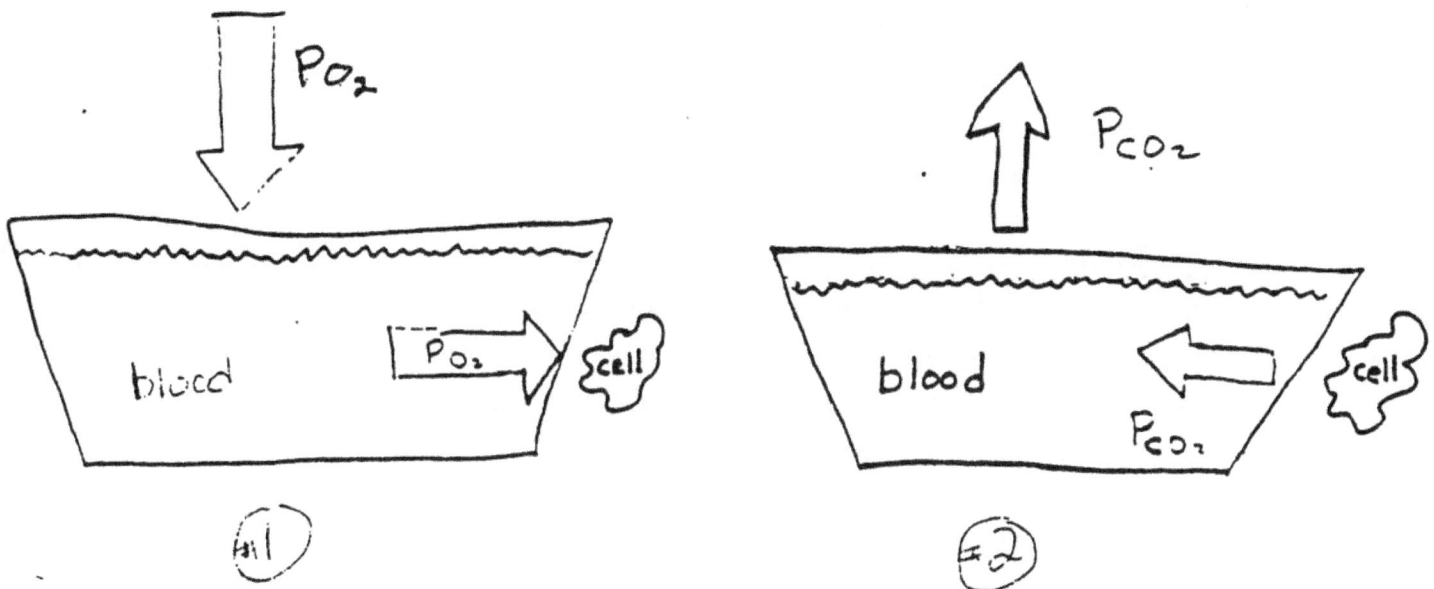

Breathing does two things. (1) It takes oxygen from the air and puts it into the blood. From the blood O_2 goes to all the cells. (2) It takes carbon dioxide from cells, through the lungs and sends it out the lungs.

O_2 goes into the blood and CO_2 goes out of the blood because of partial pressure differences. P_{O_2} is 100 mmHg in the lungs and 37 in the blood passing through the lungs. Returning venous blood has a partial pressure of 45. That's higher than 40 in the lungs.

Measuring Partial Pressure (P$_{a}$O$_2$) of
O$_2$ in blood gases and
Oxygen Saturation (O$_2$ Sat.)

The first reason for blood gases is a visible
respiratory problem. That makes sense.
What you'll frequently see before blood
gases are drawn is an oxygen saturation
level.

This is a small device that clips on the
patient's finger.

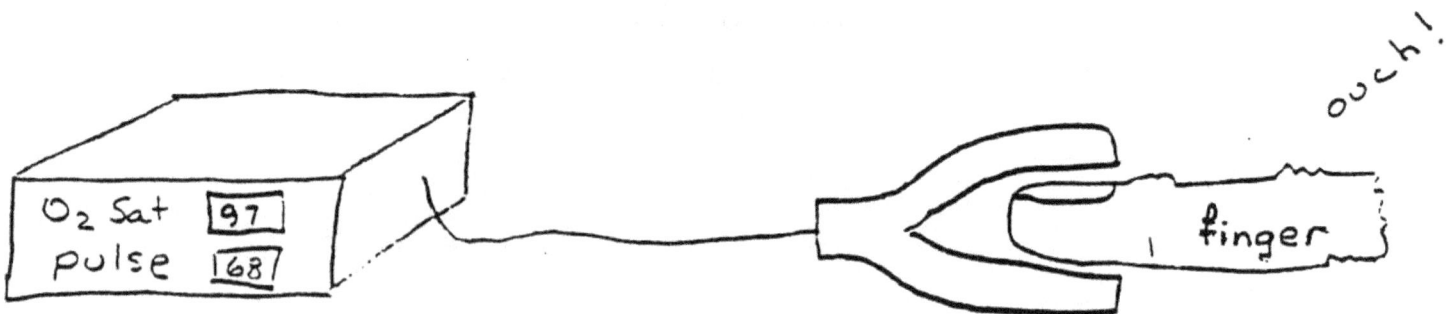

A wire connects it to a box that displays
the patients pulse and oxygen saturation
level. The oxygen saturation is the
percentage of hemoglobin that is bound to
an oxygen molecule. Hemoglobin is the
molecule in the blood that carries oxygen
to the cells. 98% O$_2$ Sat. means that 98%
of the hemoglobin is attached to an oxygen
molecule. Anything less than 90% is
probably worth looking at more closely.

A more accurate measure of oxygen levels is of course, blood gases. Here you will see the PaO_2. These are usually drawn from the radial arterial. The "a" in PaO_2 stands for arterial. For simplicity in this book, I have mostly omitted the small "a," but to be absolutely correct is should be there.

Partial pressure of oxygen in the blood is the same concept as partial pressure of oxygen in the atmosphere. You may recall that partial pressure is the pressure exerted by each individual gas in a mixture of gases. You may also remember that the atmosphere is composed almost entirely of nitrogen and oxygen. The pressure exerted by each gas is the percentage of the total volume occupied by that gas.

The total atmospheric pressure is 760mmHg. Oxygen is about 21% of atmospheric air. So the partial pressure of oxygen is 21% of 760mmHg which is about 159mmHg. The partial pressure of nitrogen is about 600mmHg. CO_2 & H_2O are less than 1%.

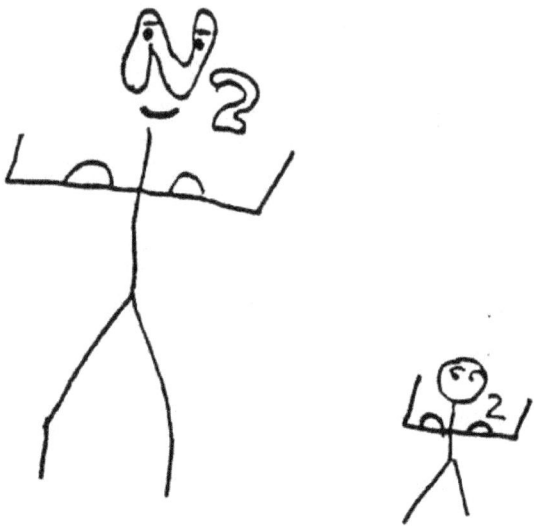

In the lungs there is more H_2O (6.2%)
& CO_2 (5.3%). Oxygen is 13.6% (104mm Hg)
and nitrogen is 74.9% (569mm Hg).

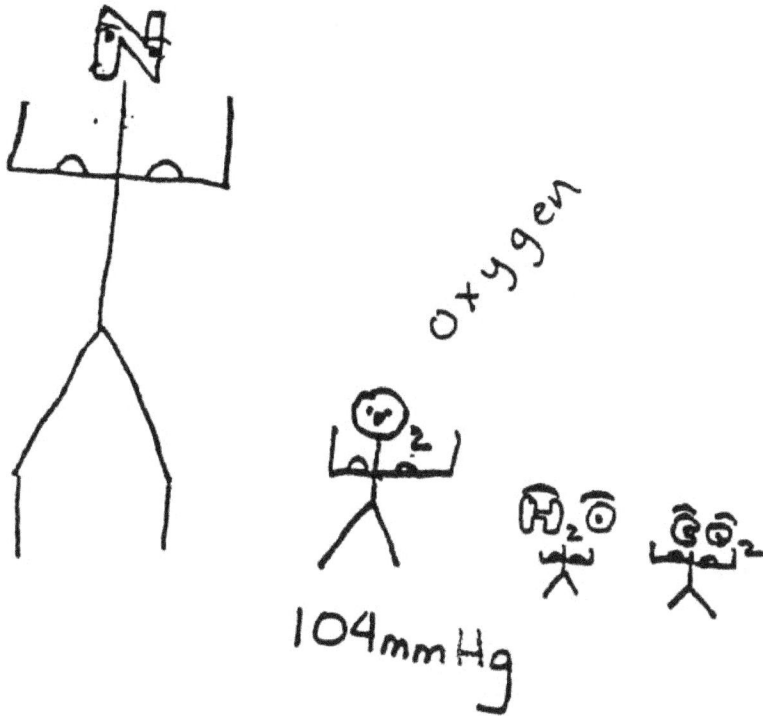

The important one here is oxygen. Blood
gases will give this partial pressure.
About 100 is normal.

WHY BREATH?

Reason #3

Breathing keeps the right H+ concentration (ph) in your body.

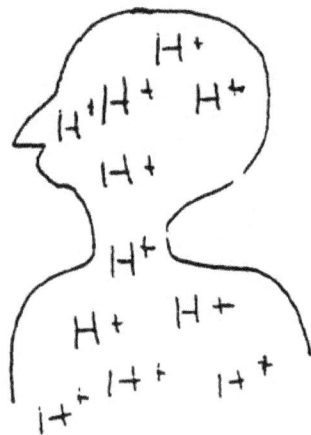

Otherwise known as respiratory control of acid-base balance.

Acid-Base Respiration

As we said earlier, the lungs act as a cleaning service to get CO_2 out of the blood.

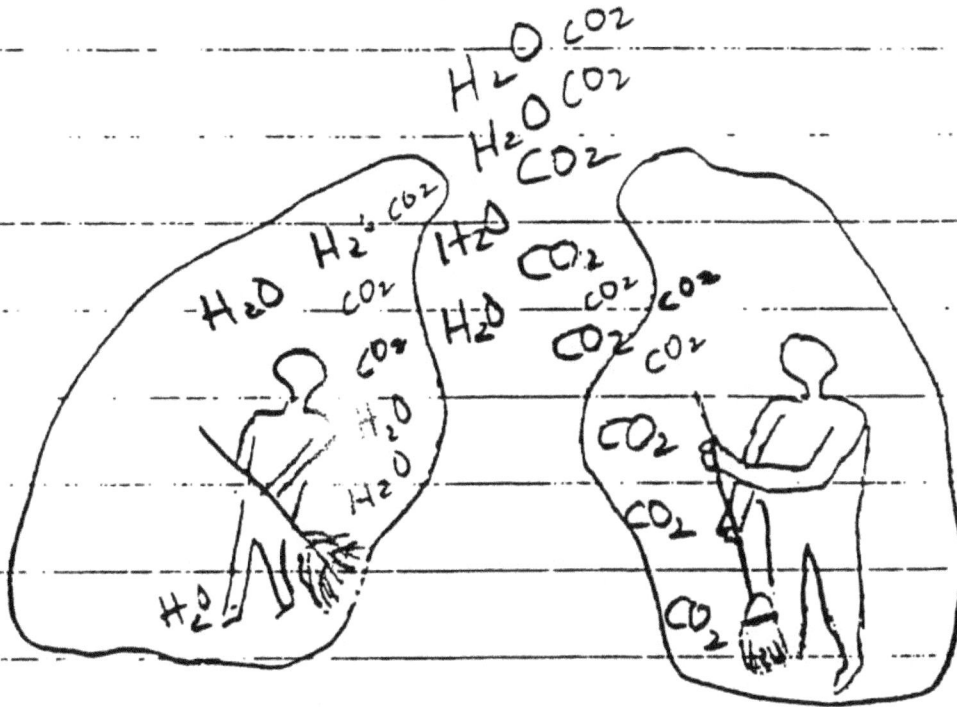

By sweeping out those two gases, it lowers the partial pressure of CO_2 & H_2O in the lungs, which allows more to diffuse from the blood.

Respiratory pH Control

Breathing maintains ph of the blood, which is the 3rd reason to breath. It does this by regulating CO_2.

Acidity is mostly caused by carbonic acid (H_2CO_3). Like any acid it throws off some H+ ions.

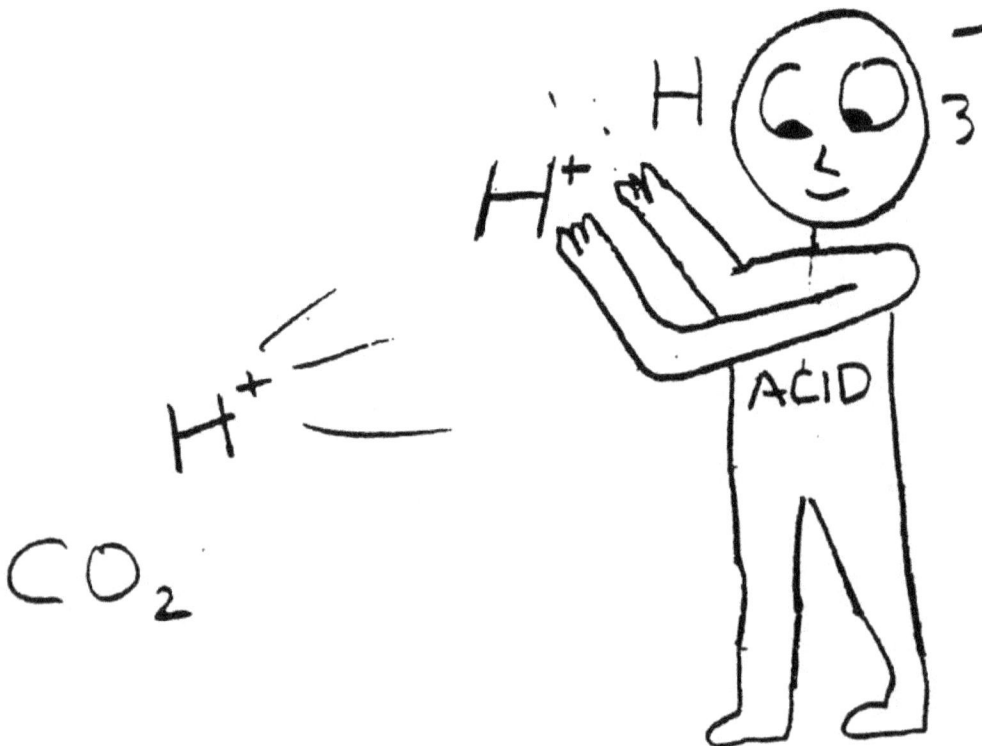

The lungs breath out CO_2 and that plucks more CO_2 out of the blood.

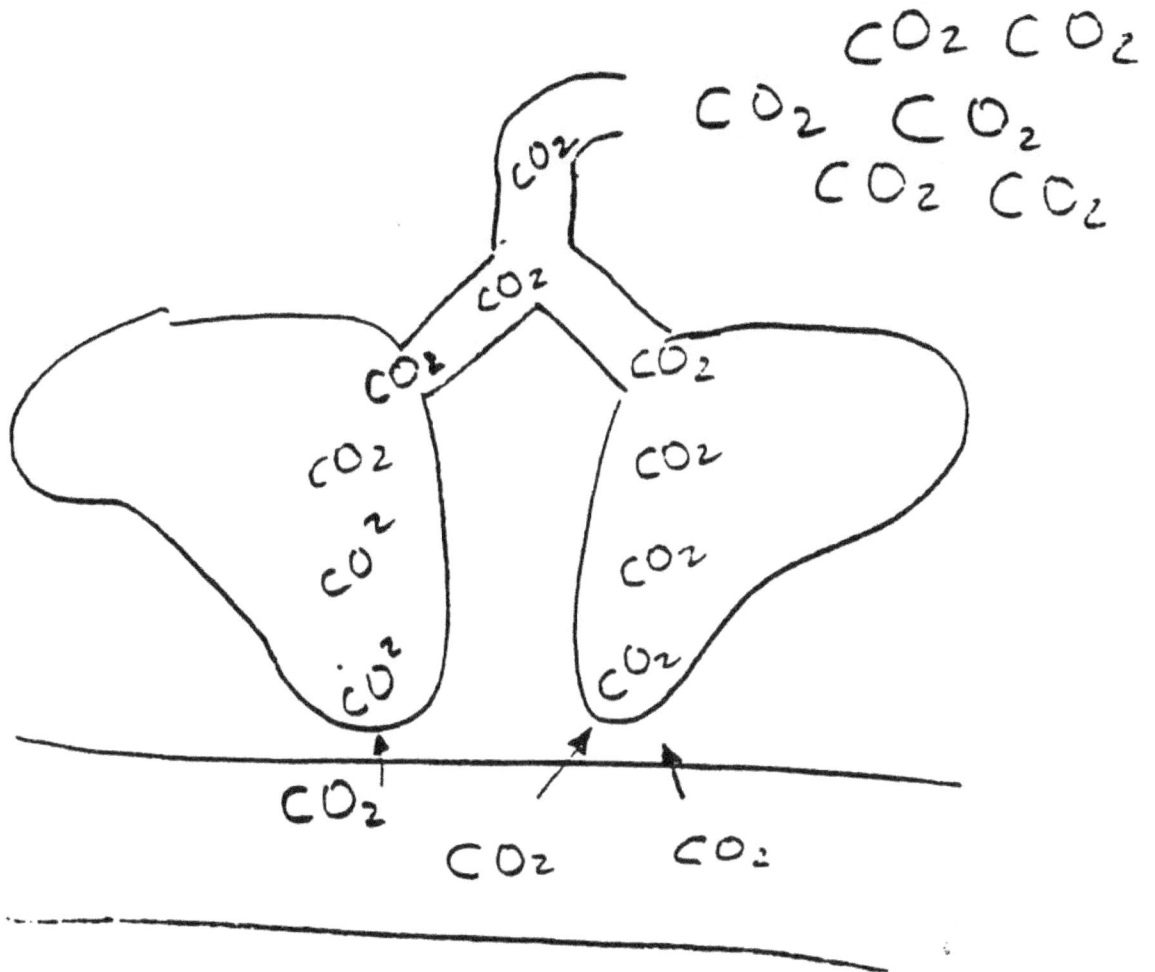

But if there isn't enough CO_2 floating around in the blood, CO_2 wants more CO_2 to swim around with.

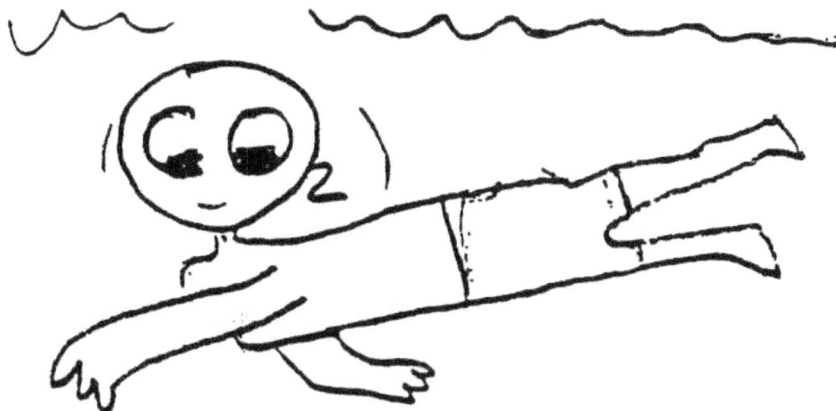

So he signals his CO_2 friends in carbonic acid to come out and play.

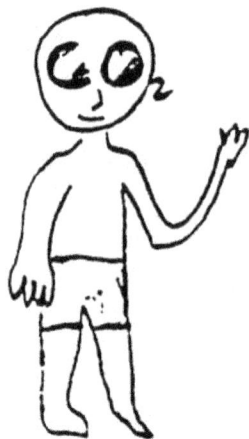

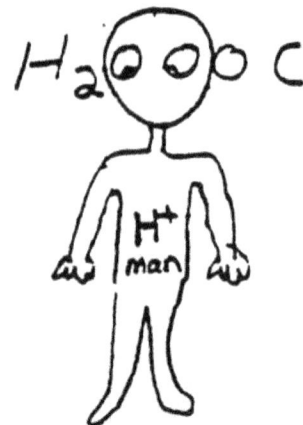

Carbonic acid just falls apart into H_2O and CO_2.

And thats how the lungs change ph and take acid out of blood.

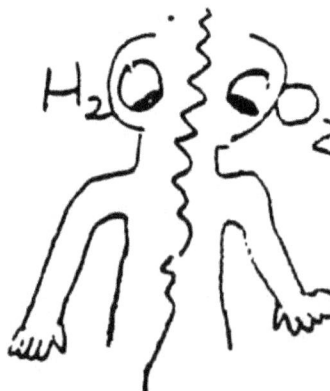

The opposite happens when the lungs let
CO_2 pile up. As we saw earlier, it will
also pile up in the blood.

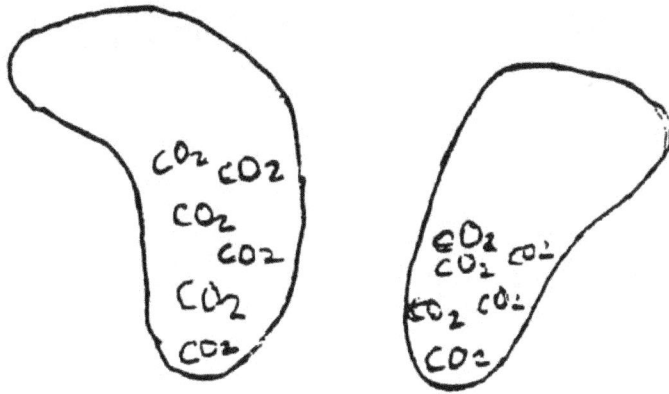

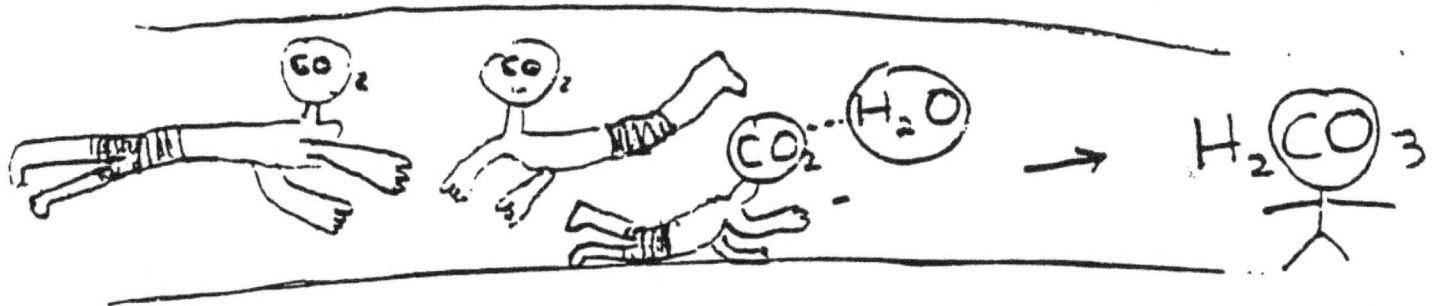

Some of the CO_2 go with their friend H_2O to
form H_2CO_3 (carbonic acid). Thats how the
lungs influence acid formation in the
lungs.

So when there is too much CO_2 in the lungs,
there is too much CO_2 in the blood. Some
of the CO_2 in the blood combines with H_2O
to form carbonic acid - which raises acidity.

Metabolic Control of ph

Other systems and processes control ph.
These are classified as **METABOLIC**.

Kidneys can raise or lower ph.

They can pump bicarb into the lungs or
cut it way back.

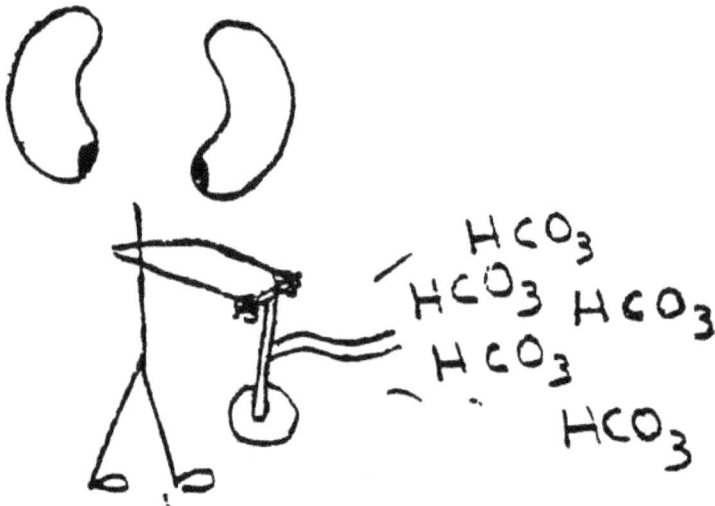

HCO_3
HCO_3 HCO_3
HCO_3
HCO_3

"no more"

metabolic
alkalosis

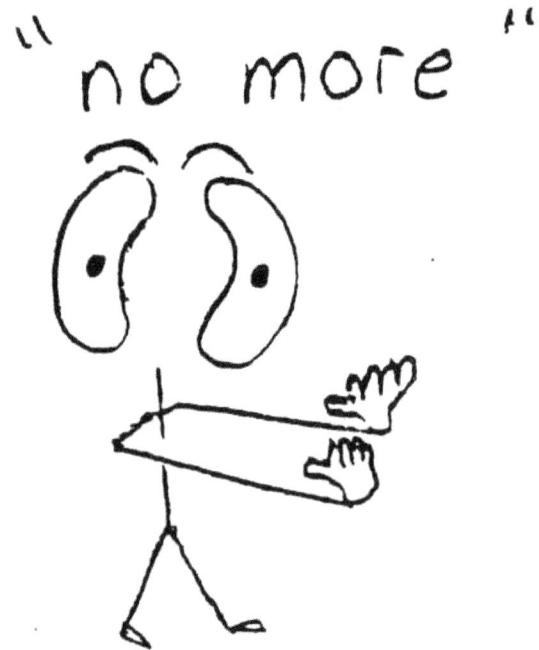

metabolic
acidosis

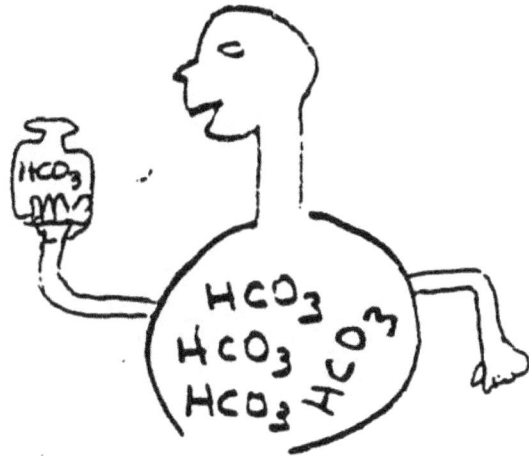

Antacids like
Tums and Maalox
contain bicarb. Too
much Maalox would cause metabolic alkalosis.

Vomitting

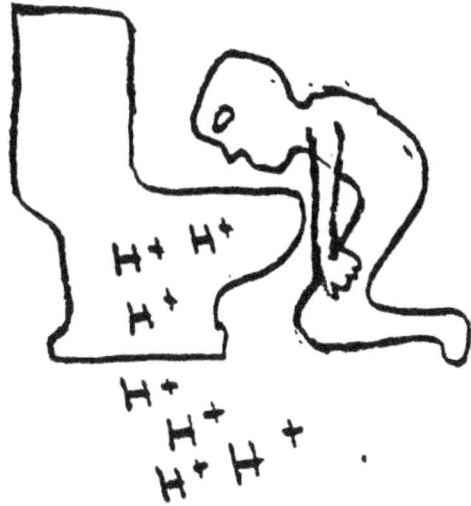

The hydrochloric
acid in your
stomach can be
vomitted into the
toilet. Losing
too many H+ would
be metabolic alkalosis.

Diabetes is a cause of acidosis. When the blood sugar goes too high and the body utilizes fats for energy Keto acids are released. The only thing you need to know is extremely high blood sugar can cause metabolic acidosis.

What Are Exactly Blood Gases?

pH

PaCO₂

PaO₂

HCO₂

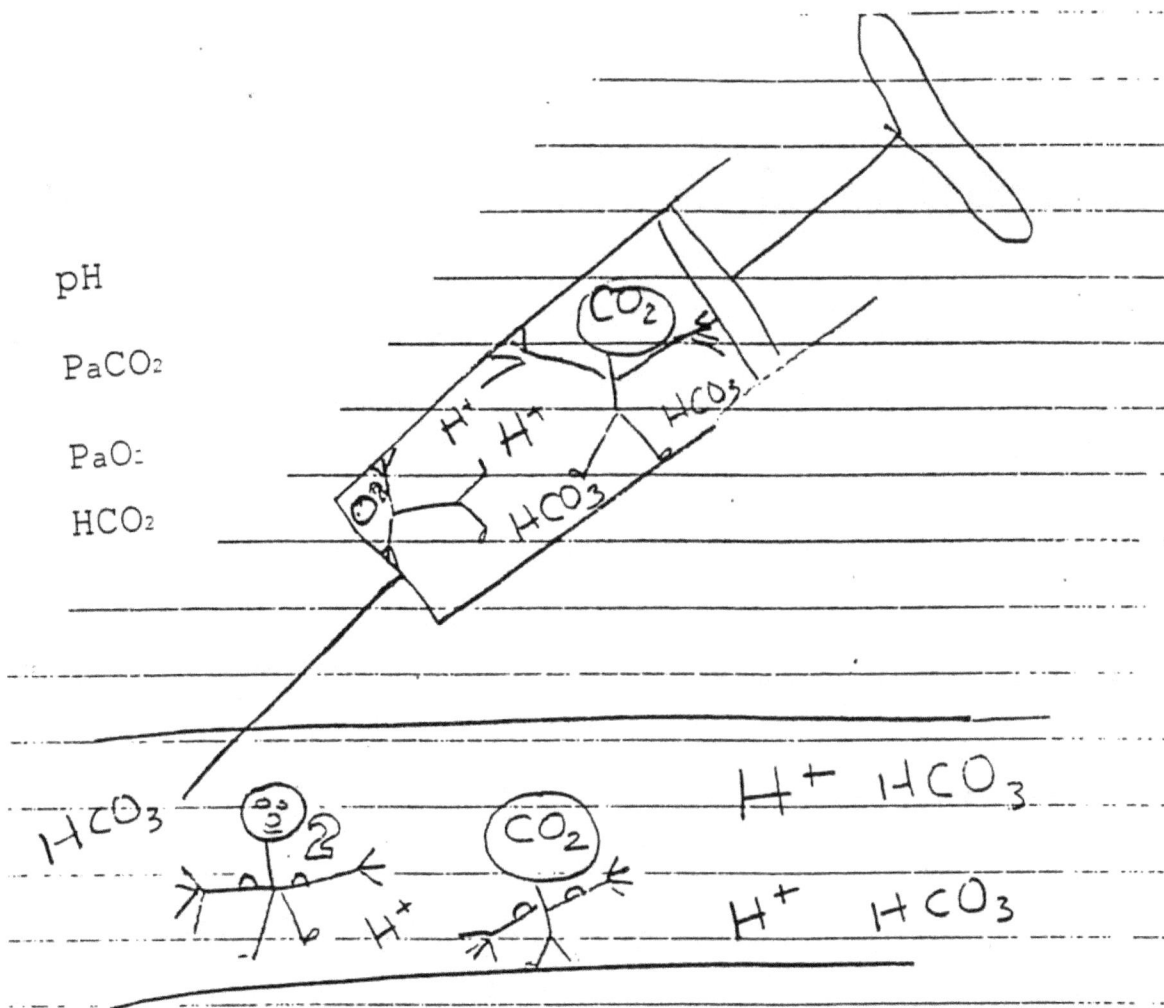

Good question.
The answer to follow - read on.

Blood gases are drawn from arteries - usually the radial. They always show:

(1) The acidity or alkalinity of the blood by the pH. Normal is 7.35-7.45

(2) The oxygenation of the blood by P_{aO_2}, partial pressure of oxygen. This value can vary a lot depending on the patients age, condition and history. Anything over 95mmHg would be okay. But values could be much lower and still be okay.

(3) Respiratory involvement. P_{aCO_2}, partial pressure of carbon dioxide, shows whether the lungs are sweeping out carbon dioxide or not. Normal values are 35-45mm Hg.

(4) Metabolic involvement. The number of bicarbonate ions floating around. 22-26 is normal.

In the blood gas section of this book
I will show these characters changing
the pH of the blood.

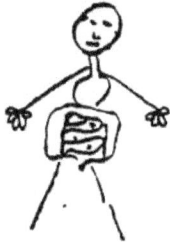

Here is metabolic causes.
You see here the stomach
and guts.

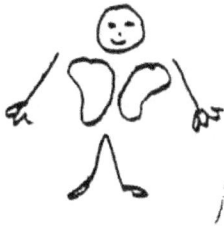

Here is respiratory causes
of pH changes. Those are
the lungs you see.

They will be pushing or pulling the
pH (which will be shown by an arrow)
on this scale.

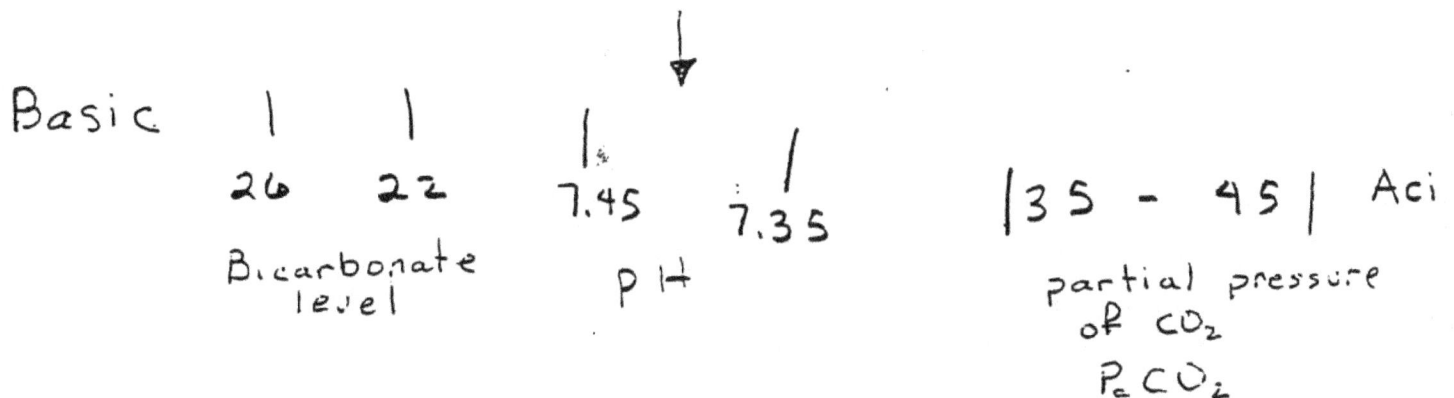

Basic

26   22   7.45   7.35 |35 - 45| Aci

Bicarbonate   pH   partial pressure
level   of CO_2
                                P_aCO_2

This picture of a tug of war illustrates ph changes and the cause.

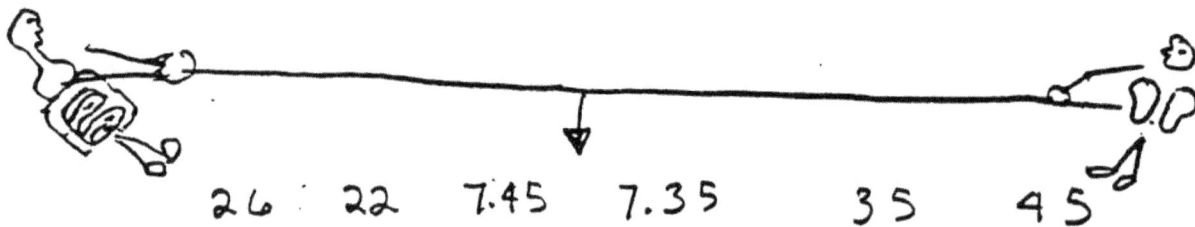

26   22   7.45   7.35   35   45

I will add this picture to all examples. Respiratory and metabolic are shown here. In this picture the lungs are pulling toward acid and metabolic is pulling toward basic.

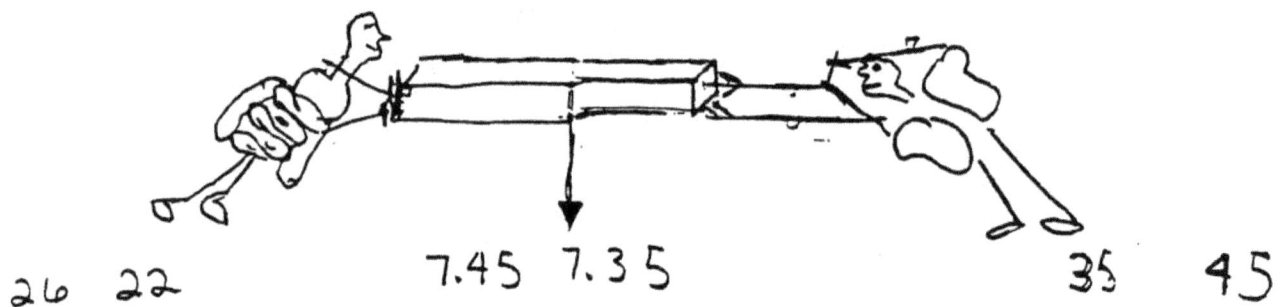

26 22   7.45 7.35   35   45

Here are the same guys (girls?) in this picture pushing. Metabolic is pushing toward acid and standing in acid (less than 22) and respiratory is standing in basic, pushing toward basic.

You can tell what the system is doing
by where the character is standing.
Normal bicard values are 22-26.
If there is too much bicarb in the blood
I have shown that as metabolic standing
past 26. He will be pulling ph toward
basic.

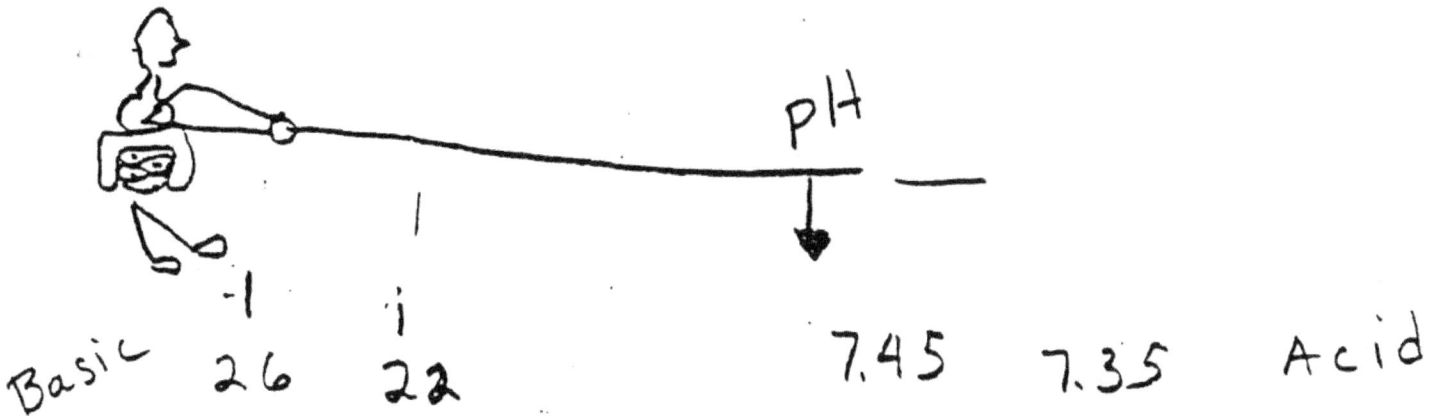

Basic   26   22   7.45   7.35   Acid

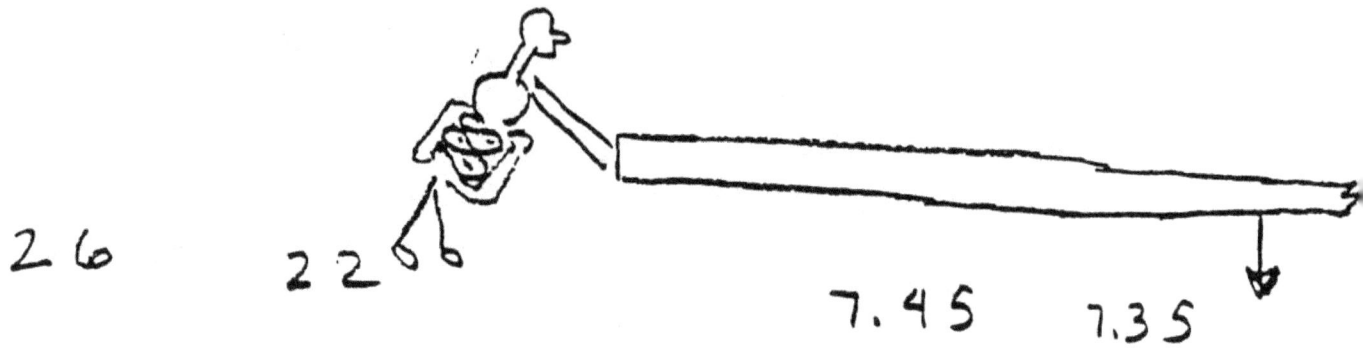

26   22   7.45   7.35

Here is metabolic with a low bicarb value
(less than 22) pushing the ph to acid levels.

The Cast in Blood Gases

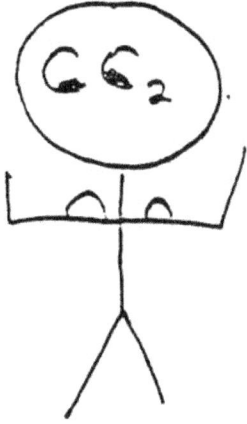

Here is the partial pressure of carbon dioxide. Notice his biceps.

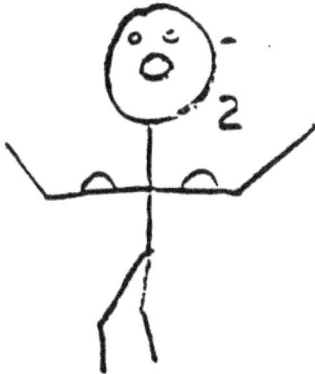

Here is the partial pressure of oxygen. Look for the chemical symbol and the biceps.

In addition to these guys, on the last page we'll use these two pushing oxygen and carbon dioxide around the system.

RESPIRATORY ACIDOSIS

All 6,000,000,000,000 cells breath out CO_2 into the blood.

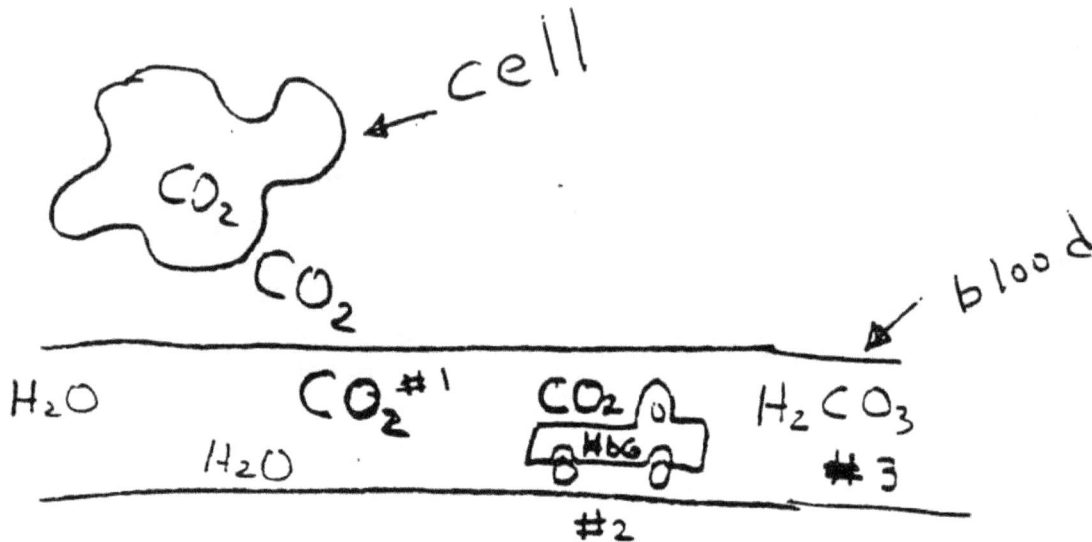

CO_2 travels three ways:

    #1.   Alone - CO_2 floating in blood

Forget #2.   Attached to Hb$_g$ (a hemoglobin
this   molecule)

    #3.   It combines with H_2O to form H_2CO
         (carbonic acid)

We are concerned with #1 and #3.

The first step in the chain of events toward respiratory acidosis is the lungs don't exhale enough carbon dioxide. There are many reasons for this. But the bottom line is that CO_2 piles up in the lungs.

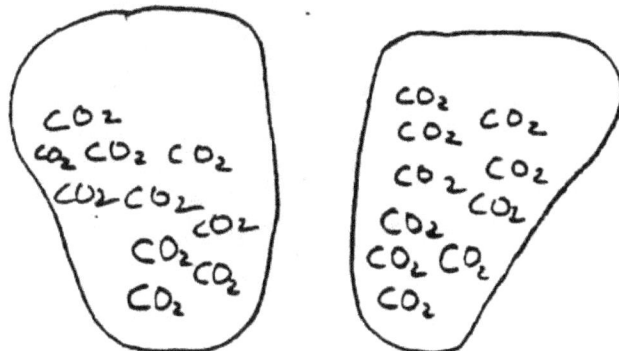

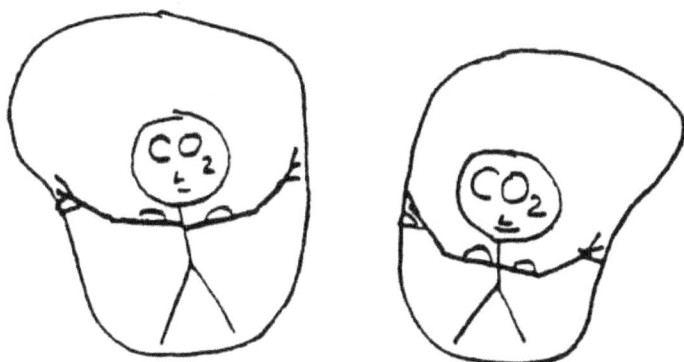

Here is the higher partial pressure of CO_2 in the lung.

If carbon dioxide builds up in the lungs, the higher partial pressure slows the diffusion of carbon dioxide <u>from</u> the blood to the lungs.

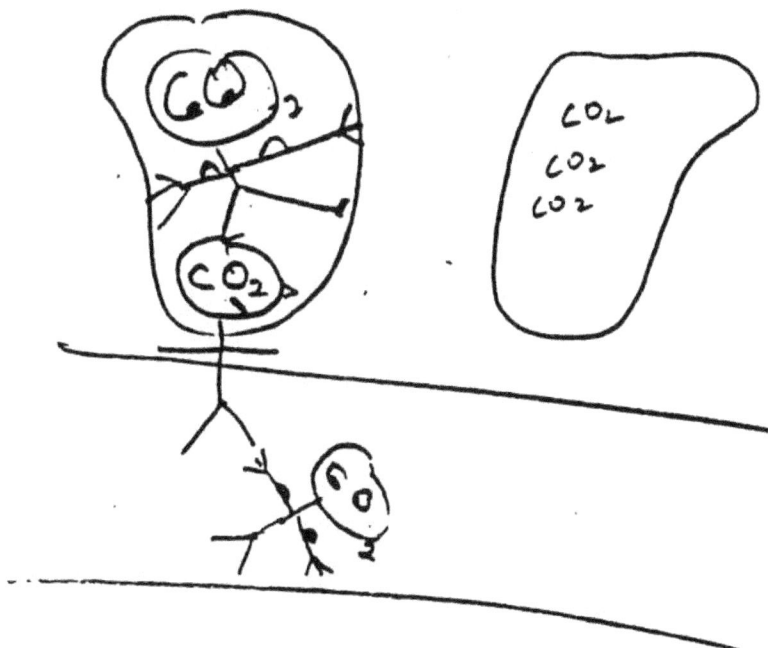

Then the CO_2 builds up in the blood.

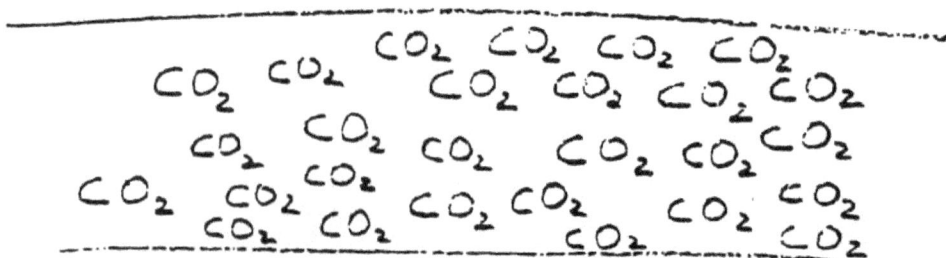

CO_2 CO_2 CO_2 CO_2 CO_2 CO_2
CO_2 CO_2 CO_2 CO_2 CO_2 CO_2 CO_2
CO_2 CO_2 CO_2 CO_2 CO_2 CO_2
CO_2 CO_2 CO_2 CO_2 CO_2 CO_2 CO_2
CO_2 CO_2 CO_2

So.... the carbonic acid which normally
splits up into H_2O and CO_2 doesn't
split up. It stays carbonic acid (H_2CO_3).

Too much carbon dioxide floating around
in the blood inhibits H_2CO_3 from breaking
up into H_2O and CO_2.

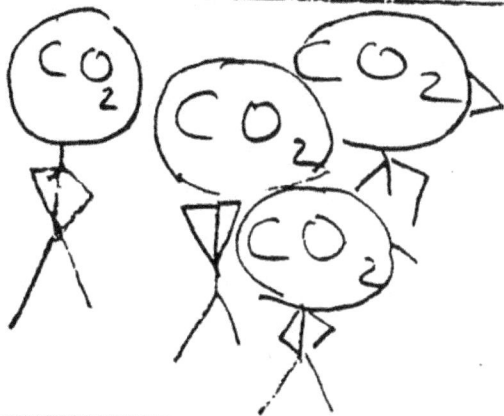
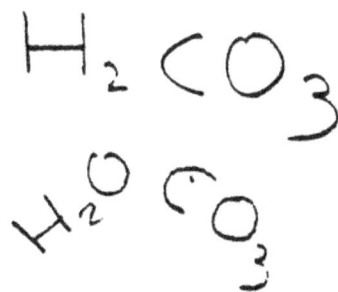

Because the carbonic acid (H_2CO_3) isn't breaking up into H_2O and CO_2 there is lots more carbonic acid. That means more acidity.

Do you see, now how more CO_2 in the lungs causes more acidity in the blood?

Here is what respiratory acidosis looks
like on our tug of war:

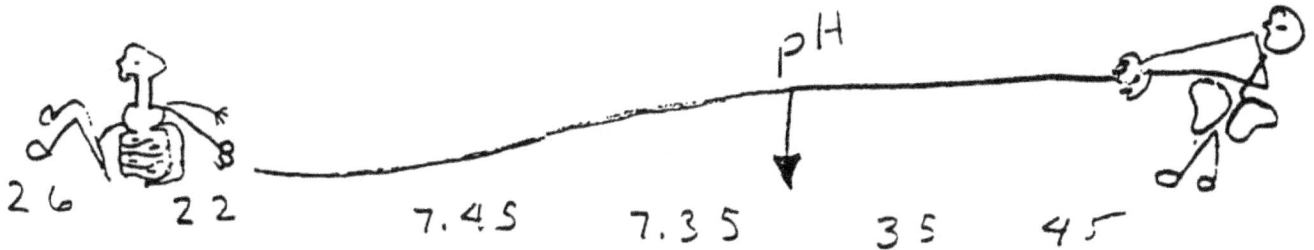

Our scale shows the lungs pulling the pH
into acid (notice where the lungs are
standing) and metabolic just sitting there.
Also notice where metabolic is sitting.

Drawing blood gases would show what the
tug of war shows.

High P_{CO_2} - greater than 45

Low pH - less than 35

Normal Bicarb - who is doing nothing unusual

Blood Gases
Measure These:

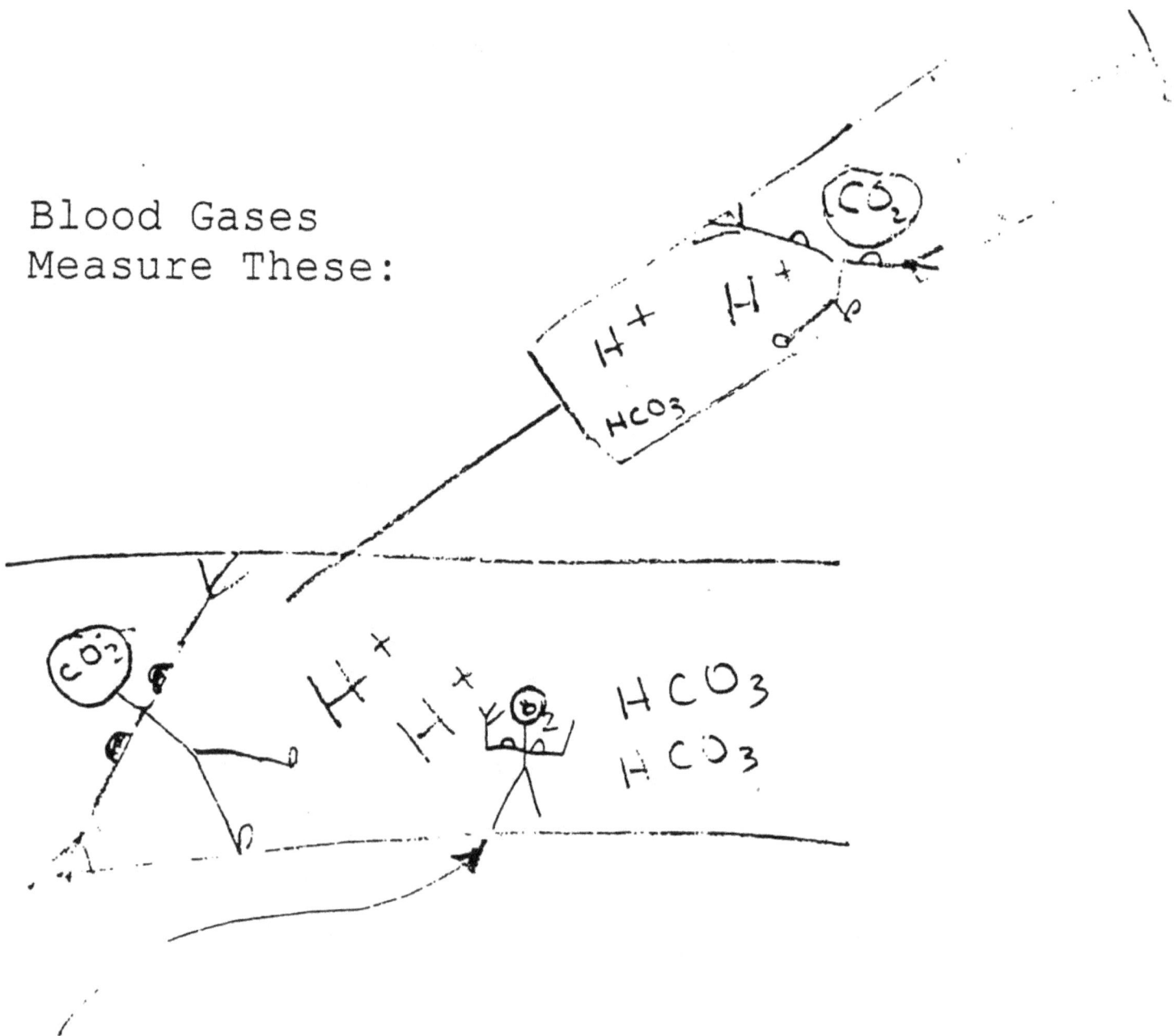

P_{O_2} is not necessarily involved. But most causes of respiratory acidosis reduce oxygenation of the blood. Things like decreased ventilation, COPD, pneumonia, severe asthma, emphysema.

Example #1

pH   7.26

P_{CO_2} 52

HCO_3 24

The first thing we look at is pH. It's low. Lots of H+ ions. Acid. The next question: How did it get this way?

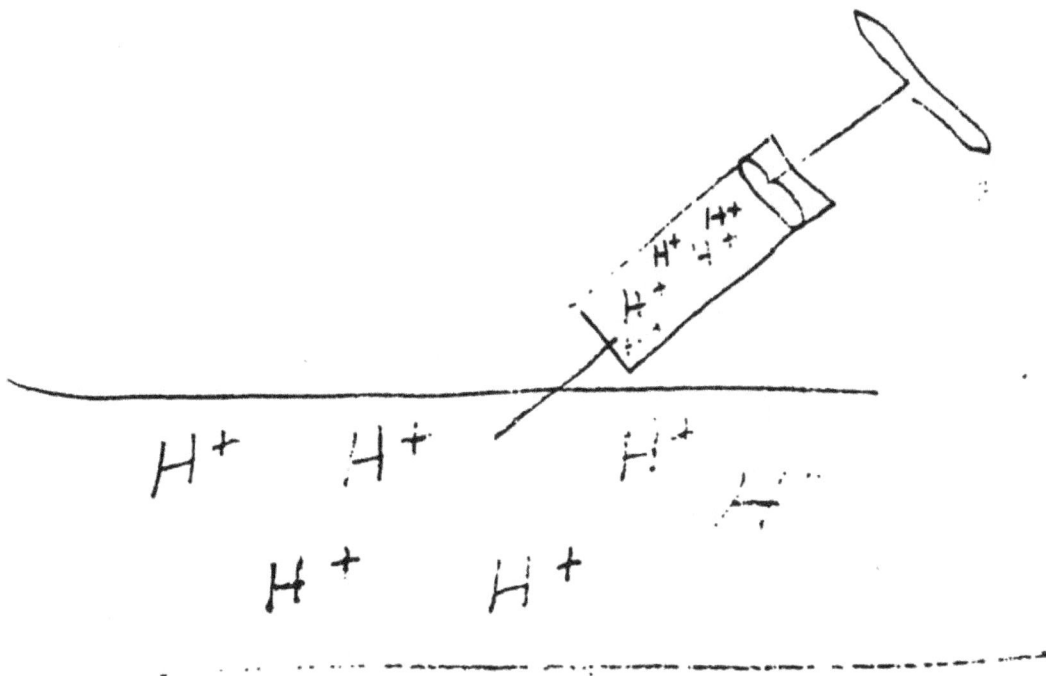

Was it because all the bicarb was lost (Diarrhea)? Or did lots of CO_2 pile up

in the lungs and then the blood. Since the
bicarb is normal, its not metabolic causes.
That leaves respiratory - which is, in fact,
who did it.

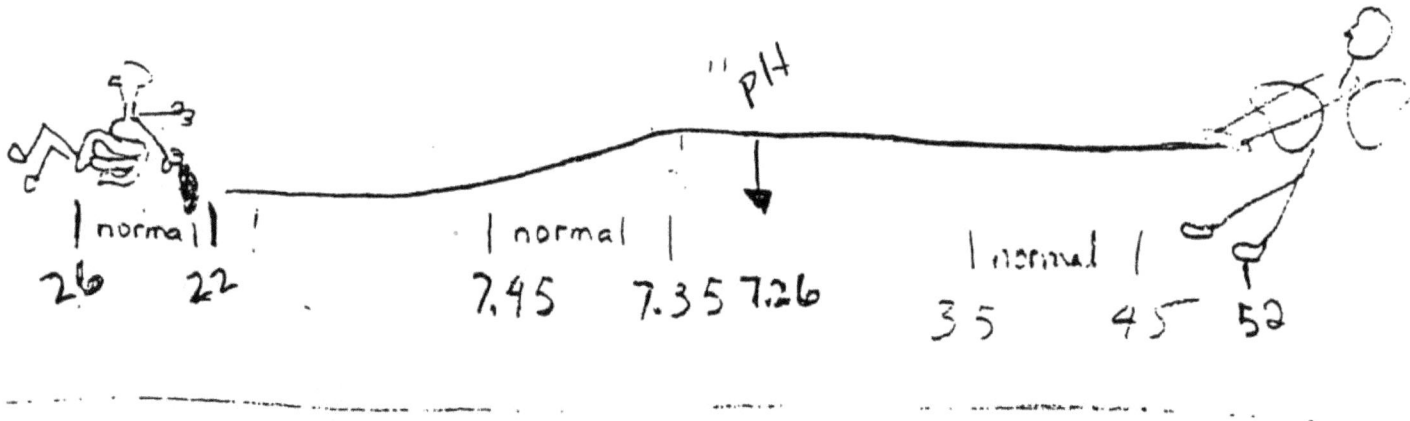

normal   normal   normal
26   22   7.45 7.35   7.26   35   45   52

Looking at our tug of war, we see the lungs
standing in acid territory pulling the pH
acid and bicarb doing nothing to stop him.

Blood gases and Turning Blue

Usually blood gases are drawn in response to signs and symptoms of poor oxygenation - changes in mental status, deep rapid breathing cyanosis. We would draw blood gases to find out why.

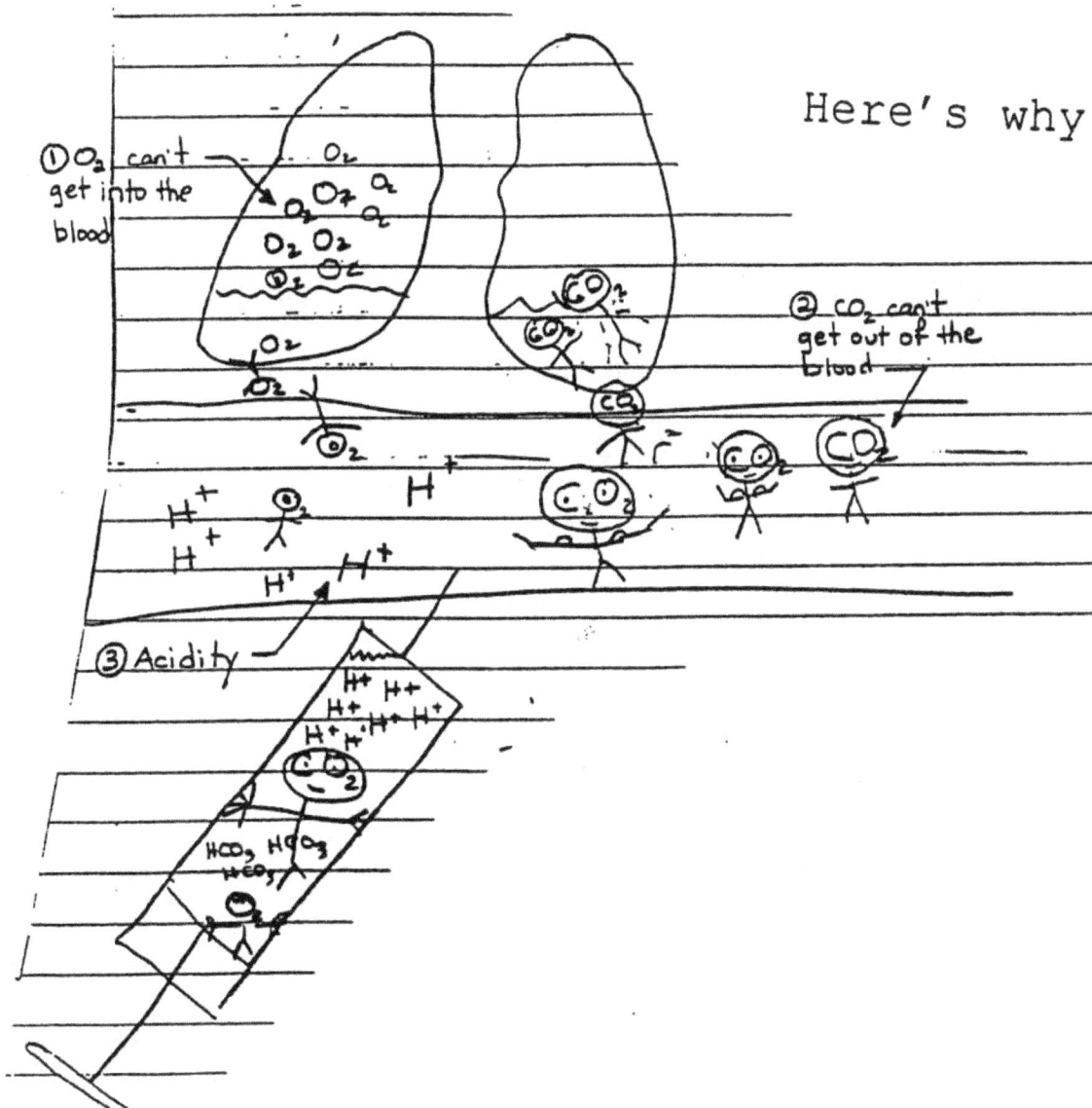

Here's why

① O_2 can't get into the blood

② CO_2 can't get out of the blood

③ Acidity

In that case of respiratory acidosis we would see:

(1) Low P_{O_2} - less than 90mmHg

(2) High P_{CO_2} - more than 45mmHg

(3) Low ph - less than 7.35

Because

(1) Oxygen can't get into the blood from the lungs.

(2) Carbon dioxide can't get into the lungs from the blood.

(3) Carbonic acid doesn't break apart. So lots of carbonic acid continues to throw off H+ ions.

Respiratory Alkalosis

Respiratory alkalosis is the opposite of respiratory acidosis. The most frequent cause is hyperventilation. Breathing very fast "blows off CO_2."

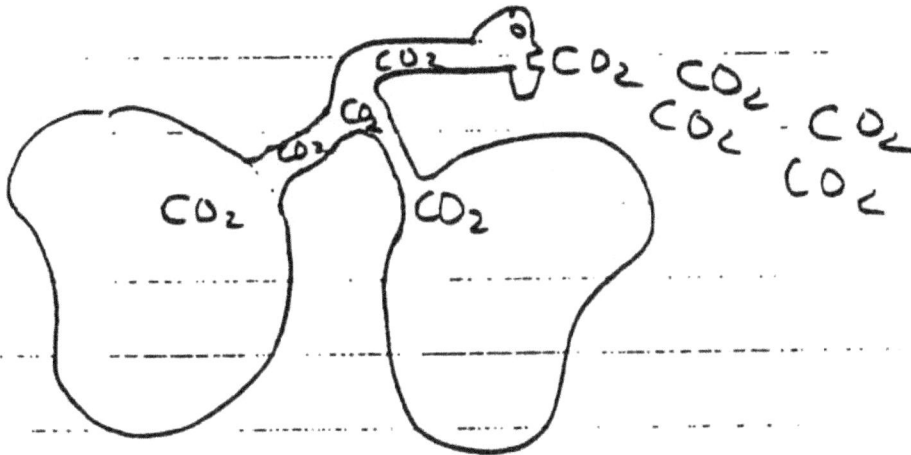

Very little CO_2 in the lungs means very little partial pressure P_{CO_2}

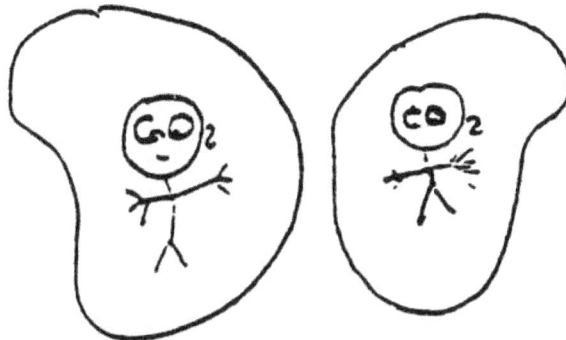

Which means very little partial pressure in the lungs to resist CO_2 escaping from the blood to the lungs.

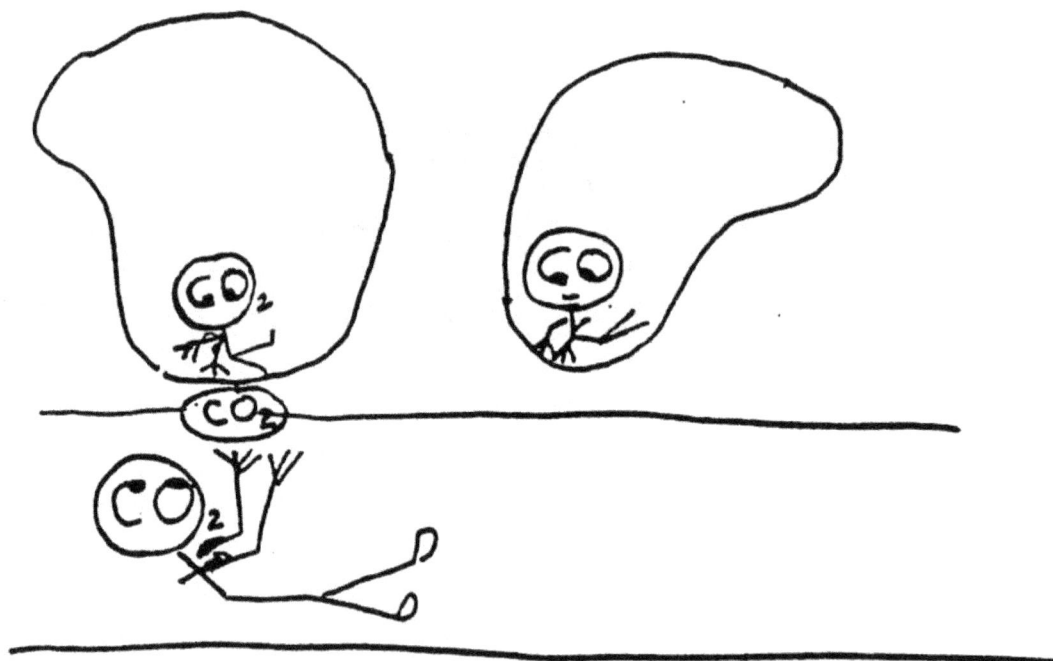

Here we see how very little P_{CO_2} in the lungs can't stop lots of CO_2 from escaping out of the blood.

Respiratory Alkalosis

If lots of CO_2 leaves the blood to the lungs....

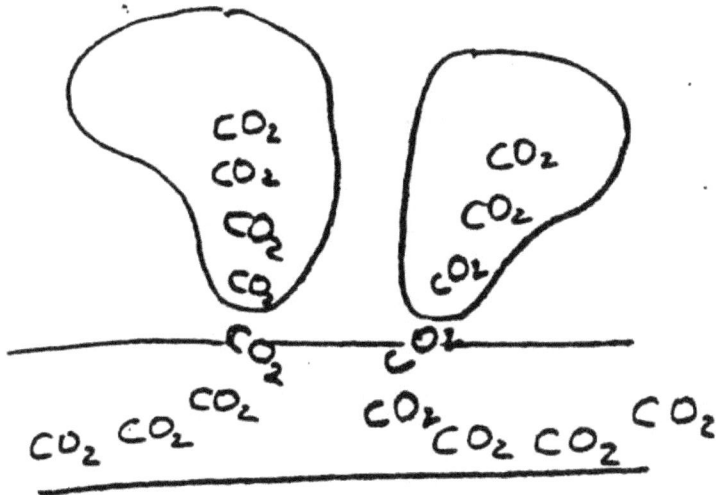

To replace the lost CO_2, carbonic acid will break down into CO_2 and H_2O.

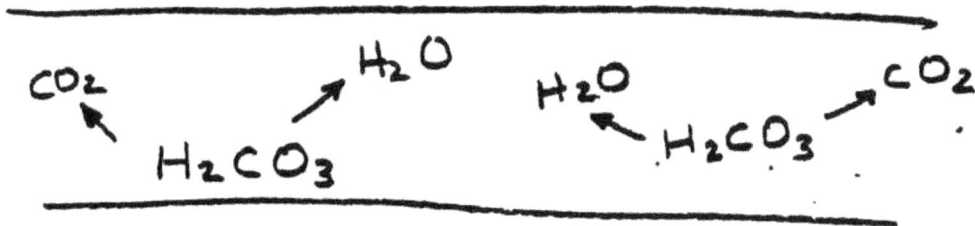

That leaves less carbonic acid which means Alkalosis.

Metabolic Acidosis

Diarrhea, diabetic ketoacidosis, renal failure, aspirin overdose, cardiac arrest (buildup of lactic acid) can cause metablic acidosis.

On blood gases this shows as:

(1) Lots of H+ ions, acid, pH less than 7.35

(2) Low bicarb, less than 22

(3) Once again, as you would expect Pco_2 nothing special

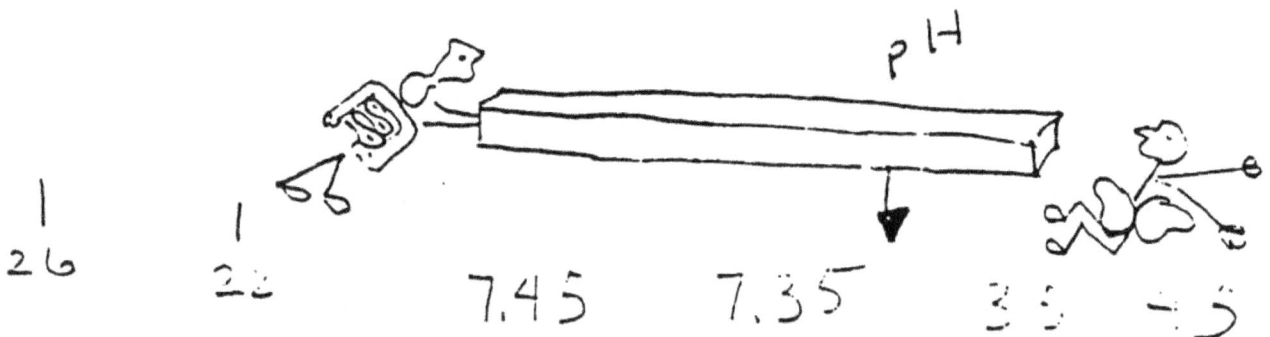

Metabolic Alkalosis

We're reviewing a little here. Excessive vomitting, too many Tums cause metabolic alkalosis.

On blood gases, this shows up as:

(1) Few H+ ions, pH greater than 7.45

(2) High bicarb, greater than 26

(3) Nothing special on P_{CO_2}

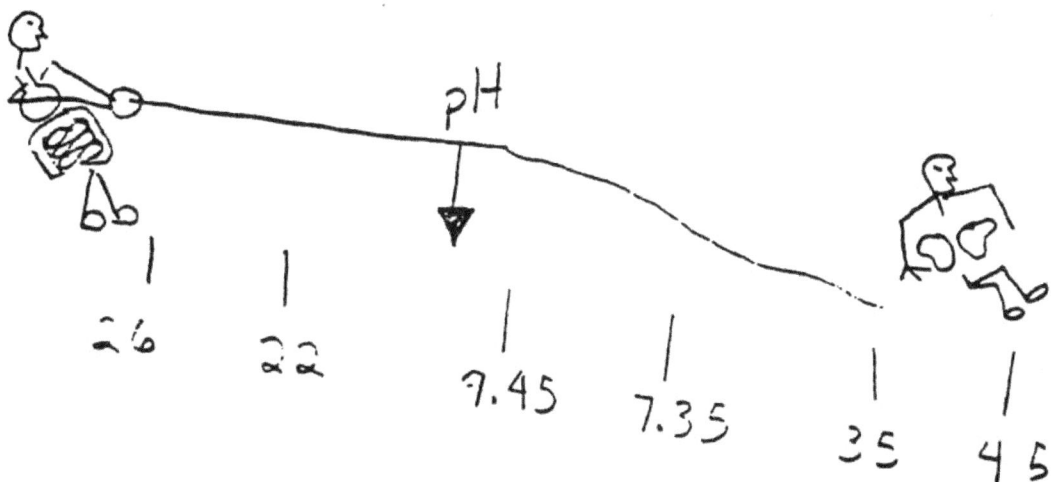

How to Approach ABG's

We just went over respiratory alkalosis and respiratory acidosis.

I have deliberately put the next section, "How to approach ABG's" after that detailed explaination.

Here are the steps you will use to determine the type and cause of blood gas abnormality:

#1.   Is the pH high or low?

#2.   Why is it too high or too low? Look on the next page to see that on a flow chart.

How to Approach Blood Gases

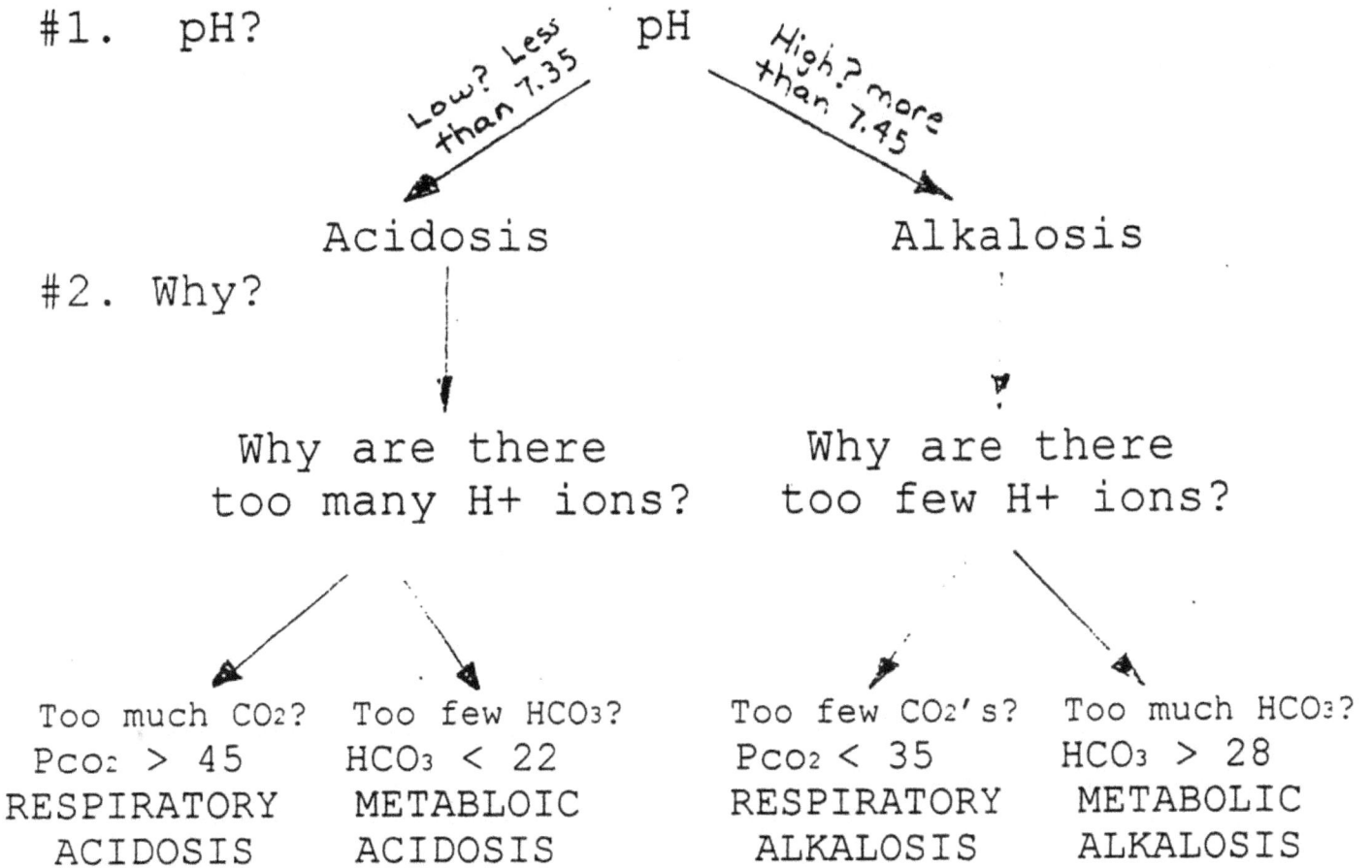

#1.   pH?   pH

Low? Less than 7.35   High? more than 7.45

Acidosis   Alkalosis

#2. Why?

Why are there
too many H+ ions?

Why are there
too few H+ ions?

Too much CO_2?	Too few HCO_3?	Too few CO_2's?	Too much HCO_3?
$P_{CO_2} > 45$	$HCO_3 < 22$	$P_{CO_2} < 35$	$HCO_3 > 28$
RESPIRATORY	METABLOIC	RESPIRATORY	METABOLIC
ACIDOSIS	ACIDOSIS	ALKALOSIS	ALKALOSIS

Example #1

Your patient is brought into the emergency
room following a motor vehicle accident.
She sustained no injuries but is extremely
upset and anxious. She has been breathing
rapidly since the crash and now feels
faint. Her ABG results are pH 7.50,
$PaCO_2$ 29, HCO_3 23.

Since the pH is definitely alkaline, there
are not enough H+ ions. Why not?

Is it because of the lungs (respiratory)?
Or is it because of the rest of the body
(metabolic)?

The bicarb level is normal (22-26) so the
cause must be respiratory.

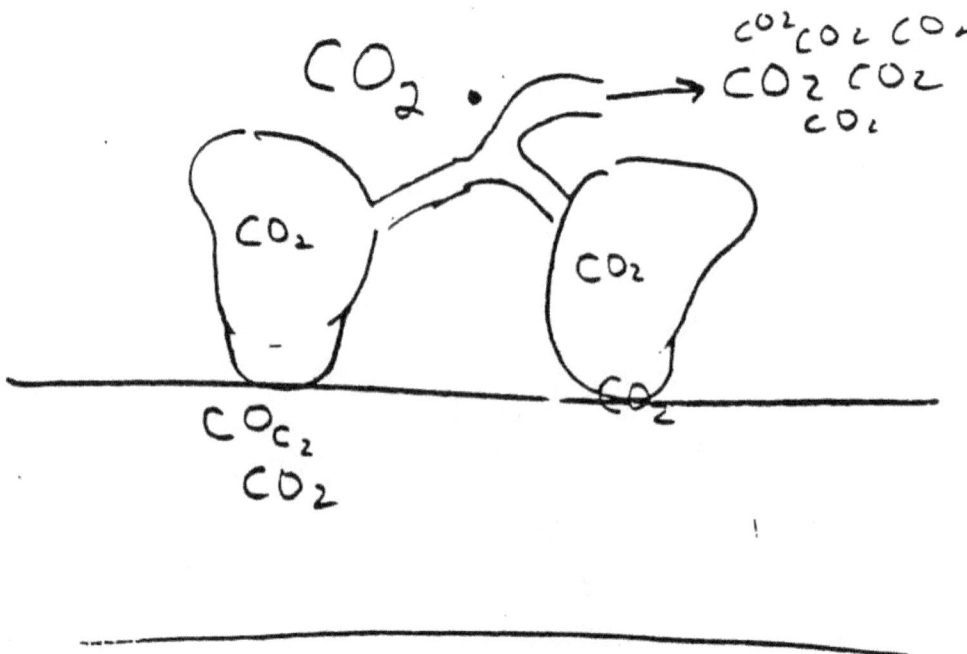

The low P_{CO_2} means CO_2 is escaping in large quantities into the lungs (where it is being "blown off"). Do you remember she's hyperventilating? The pH is high (alkalotic, too few H+) because there isn't enough CO_2 and the carbonic acid keeps breaking down into H_2O and CO_2, so there's less carbonic acid.

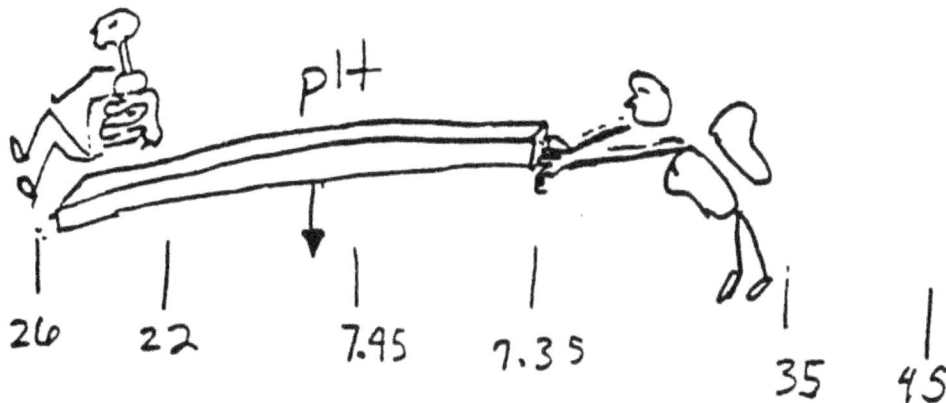

Here we see the lungs pushing (from low CO_2) the pH to alkalosis and metabolic is doing nothing to stop him.

Example #2

```
pH      7.55
Pco₂    40
HCO₃    32
```

1ˢᵗ Question: Acid or Alkalosis?
pH is high. That's alkalotic. Few H+ ions.

2ⁿᵈ Question is WHY?
Pco₂ is normal. Bicarb is High.

That means the bicarbonate ions are grabbing
the H+ ions and lowering the number of
free H+ ions floating around. That raises
the pH. Metabolic Alkalosis.

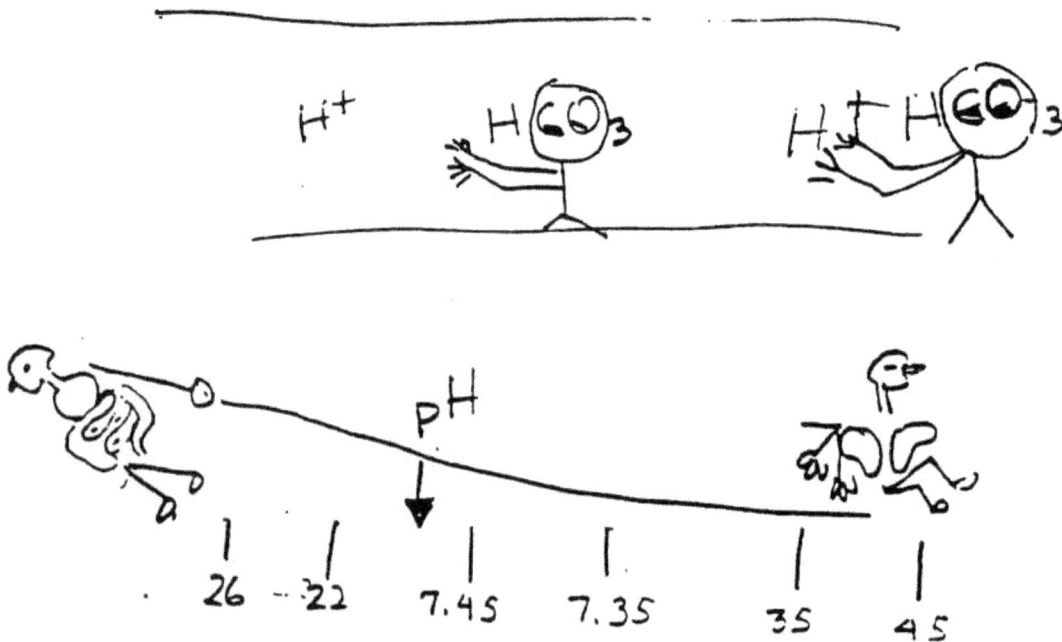

Example #3

You patient has smoked three packs a day for 40 years and is coughing up green sputum and is short of breath. His ABG results are pH 7.25, Pco_2 52, HCO_3 26. This example should be pretty obvious.

#1.   The pH is low (normal 7.35 to 7.35)
       Too many H+ floating around

#2.   Why? Is it respiratory or metabolic?
       The bicarb level is normal (22-26),
       the Pco_2 is high (normal 35-45), so
       too much CO_2 is floating around and
       that means the excess CO_2 is causing
       the acidosis.

Example #3

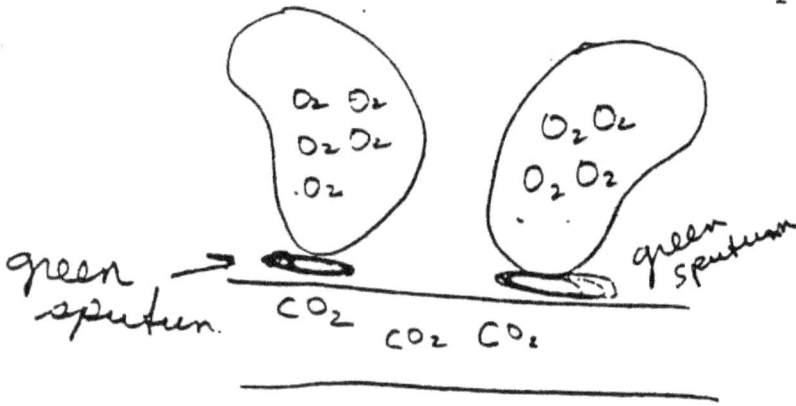

Because of the green sputum and damaged lungs (from smoking) CO_2 can't escape from the blood into the lungs. Also, O_2 can't get from the lungs into the blood.

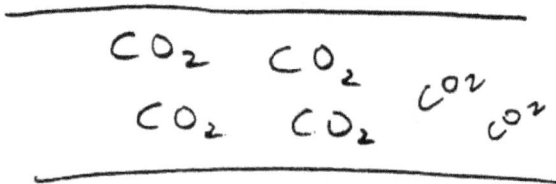

CO_2 builds up in the blood. High CO_2 levels like 52.

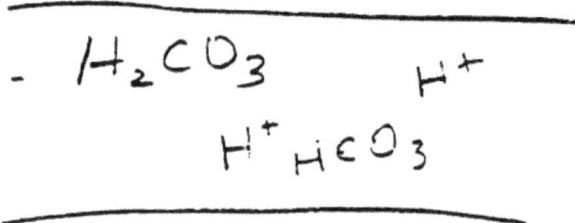

Carbonic acid doesn't break down so the blood becomes acidotic - Respiratory acidosis.

This is probably the best example of blood gases to determine the cause.

Compensation

"Compensated" means that the lungs or kidney's try to straighten out the pH problem which they didn't cause.

Metabolic compensation is the kidney's trying to raise or lower the bicarb as needed (when the lungs cause the problem).

Respiratory compensation is the lungs raising or lowering CO_2 as needed when the rest of the body caused the problem.

Full compensation means the lungs or kidneys brought the pH to normal limit (7.35 - 7.45).

Partial compensation means the lungs or kidneys didn't quite get the pH back to normal - almost. Usually 7.33 - 7.34 or 7.46 - 7.47.

The main way to spot compensation is the pH normal or close to normal and the PCO_2 and bicarb way off.

Respiratory Acidosis with
Metabolic Compensation

If the blood is too acetic the pH is low, below 7.35, too many H+ ions in solution.

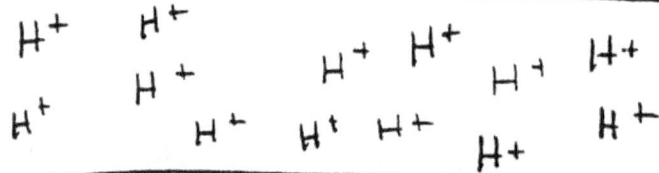

The kidney compensates by secreting bicarbonate to take out some of the excess H+.

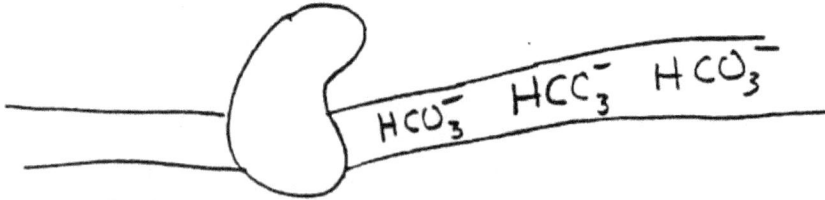

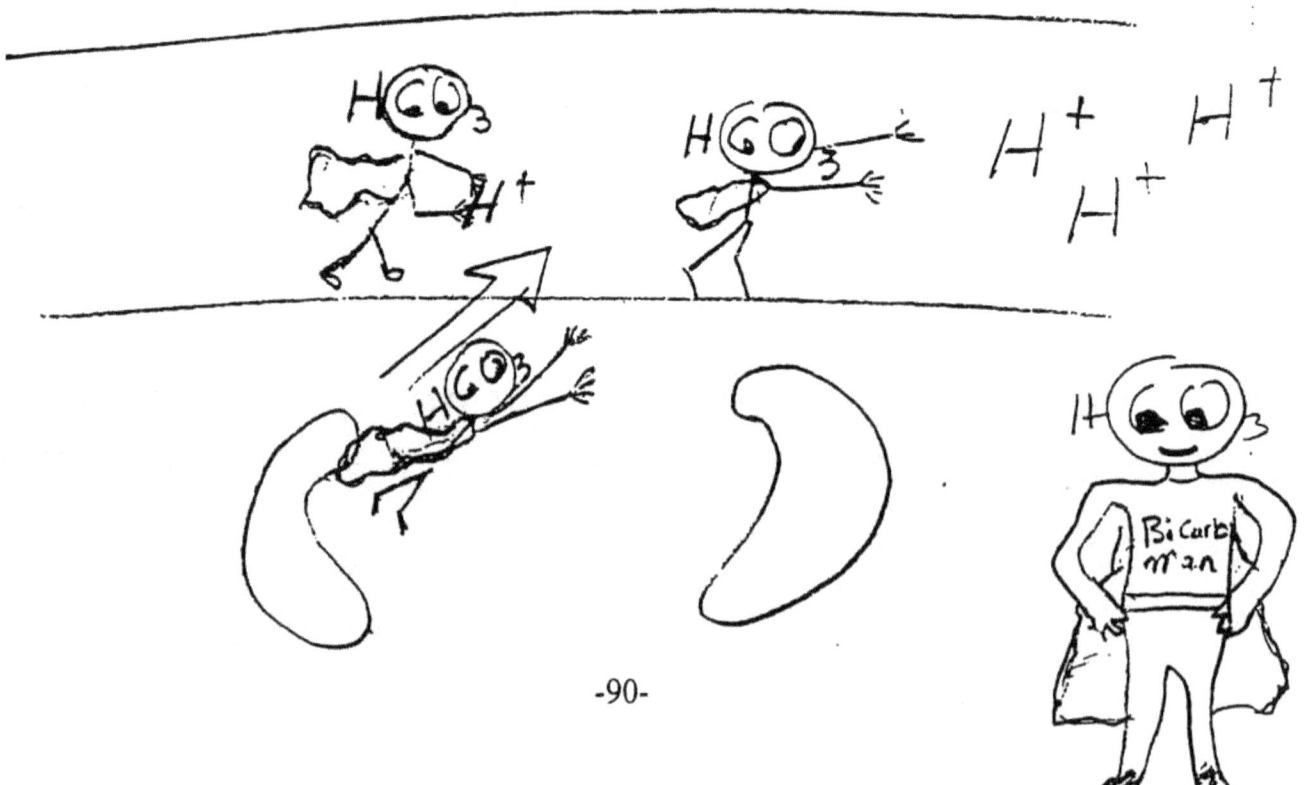

-90-

Metabolic Compensation
How it Works

The sudden windfall of bicarbonate $H_3O_3^-$ grabs all the extra $H+$, thereby bringing down the acidity, (or the pH goes up).

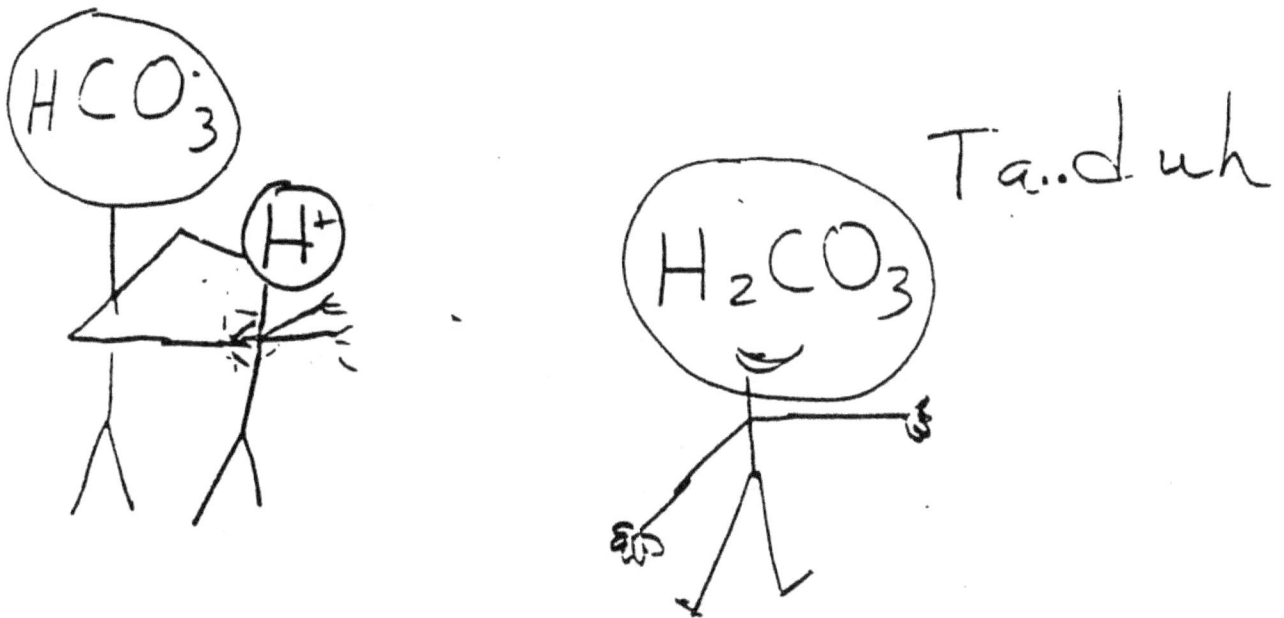

It is this ability to add bicarbonate to the blood that is the kidney's main role in acid base balance.

How You Can Tell When The Kidney is Compensating

What you would see on blood gases. If the pH is normal or close to normal and <u>large</u> amounts of bicarb

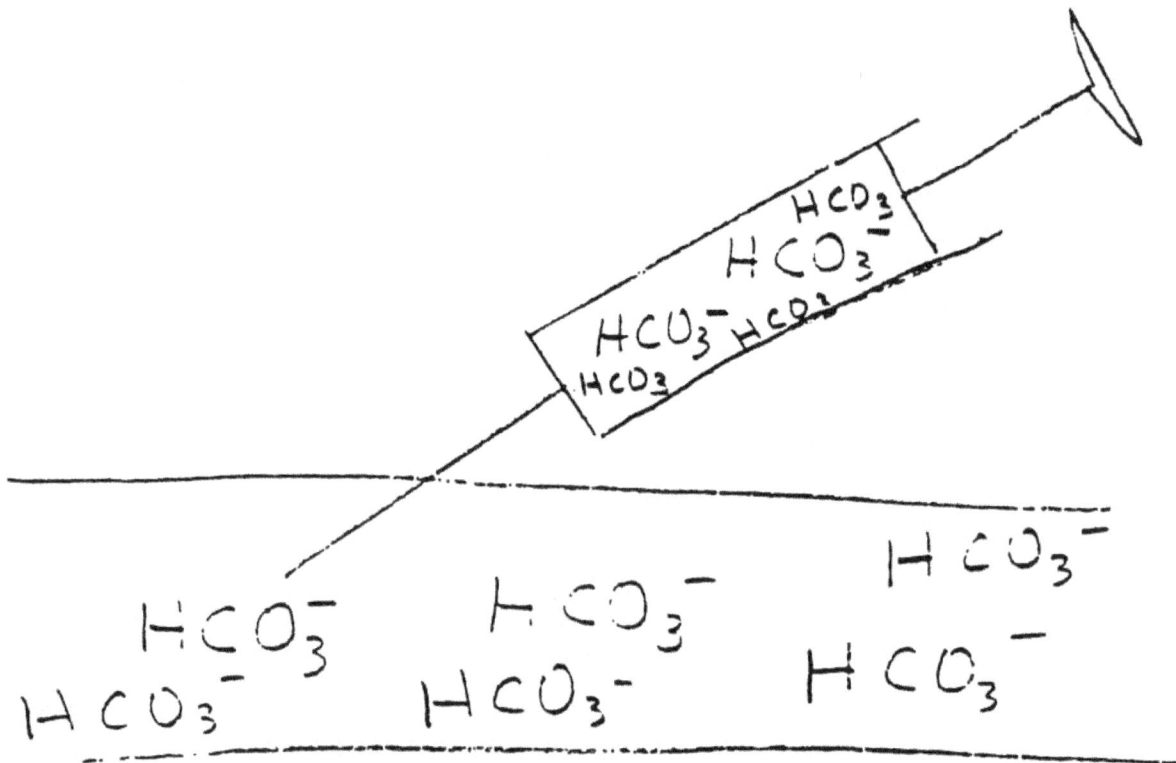

<u>Large</u> amounts of "bicarb" means the kidney is compensating for something.

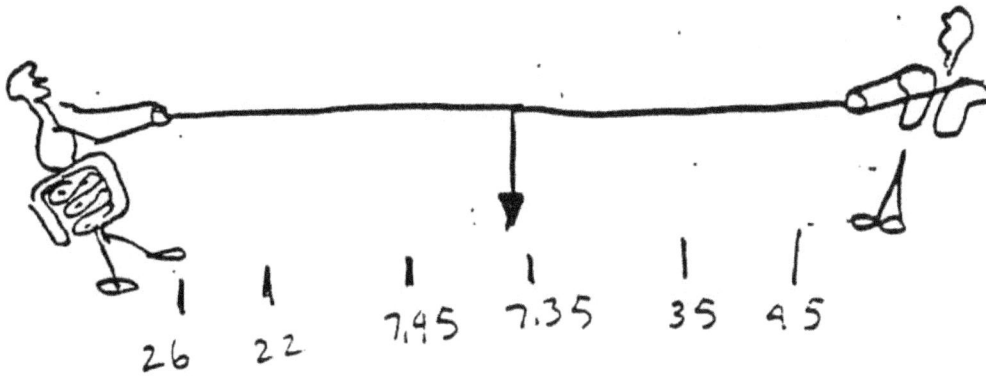

Here we have it sports fans

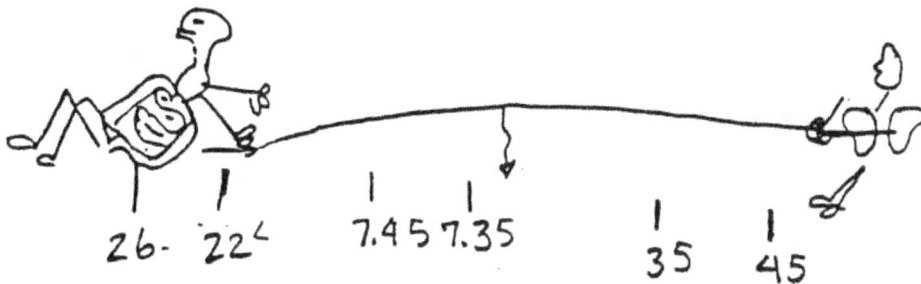

First the lungs pull the pH into acid
territory. Then the kidneys spring into
action and pump bicarb for metabolic
compensation.

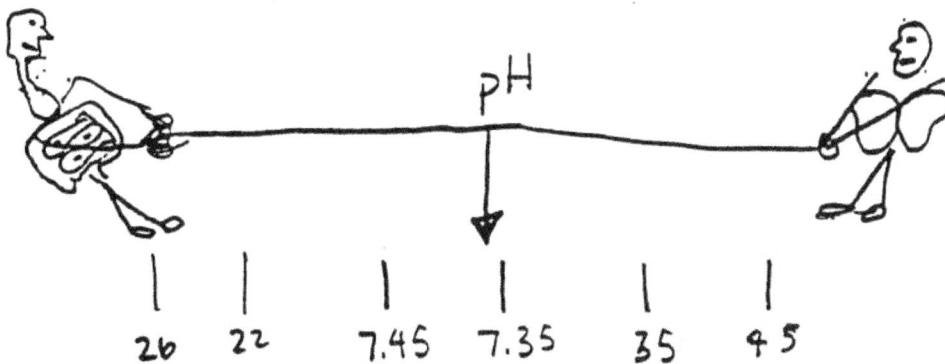

This is the typical respiratory acidosis
with metabolic compensation, pH very close
to acid, CO_2 pulling toward acid and bicarb
wide open pulling the other way.

If the metabolic compensation didn't quite make it - didn't quite get the pH to normal. It only missed it by a little.

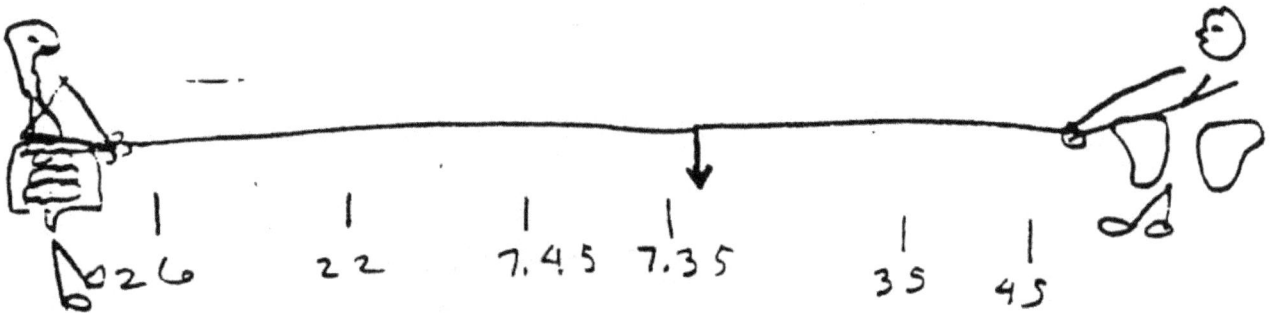

That's partial compensation. So a pH of 7.33 would be partial metabolic compensation and a pH of 7.36 would be full metabolic compensation.

Respiratory Alkalosis With
Metabolic Compensation
(just the opposite)

If there aren't enough H+ ions in the
blood, the kidneys can withhold bicarb.
that means fewer pesky bicarbs to sneak
up on and grab H+ ions.

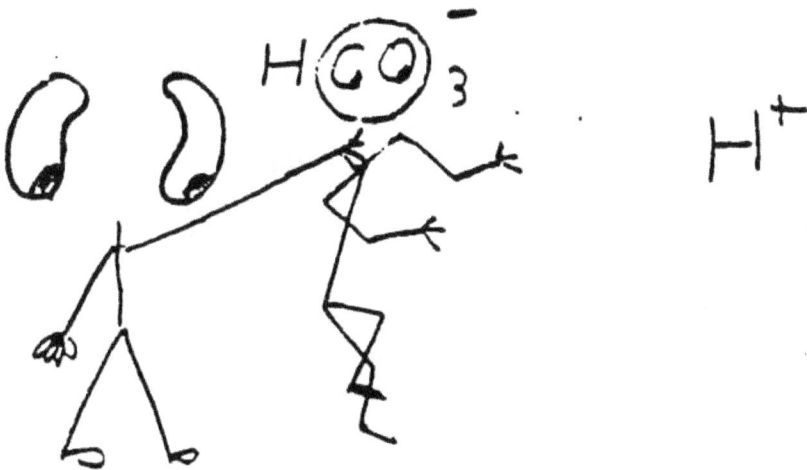

That would be called respiratory alkalosis
with metabolic compensation, which is just
the opposite, right?

On blood gases that would show up as:

pH high - but still within normal limits - about 7.44

PCO_2 - low - the cause alkalosis

Bicarb - very low - less than 21 - to the rescue

Extremely <u>low</u> amounts of bicarb mean the kidney is compensating by withholding bicarb.

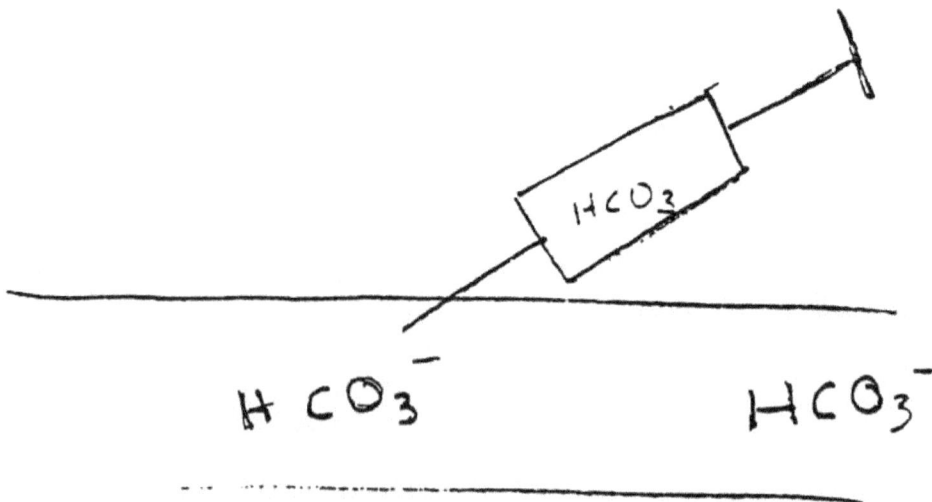

Respiratory Alkalosis With
Metabolic Compensation

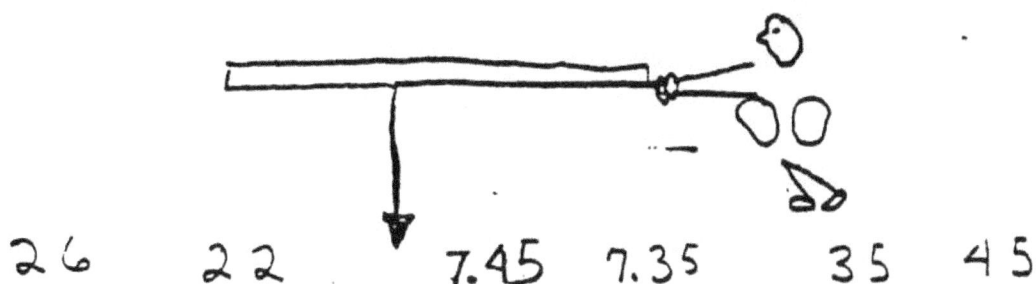

26   22   7.45 7.35   35   45

First the lungs push the pH into basic,
more than 7.45.

Then the kidneys spring into action and
withhold bicarb. Notice bicarb below 22
driving the pH back.

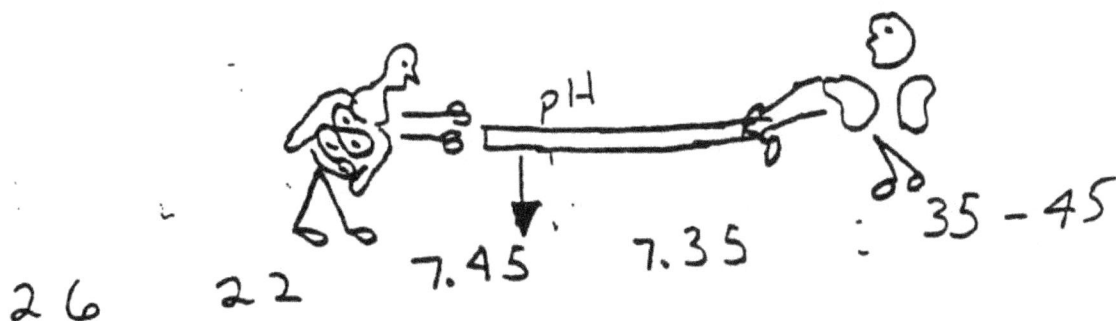

26   22   7.45   7.35   35 - 45

That would be respiratory alkalosis with
FULL metabolic compensation because it
got the pH back to normal.

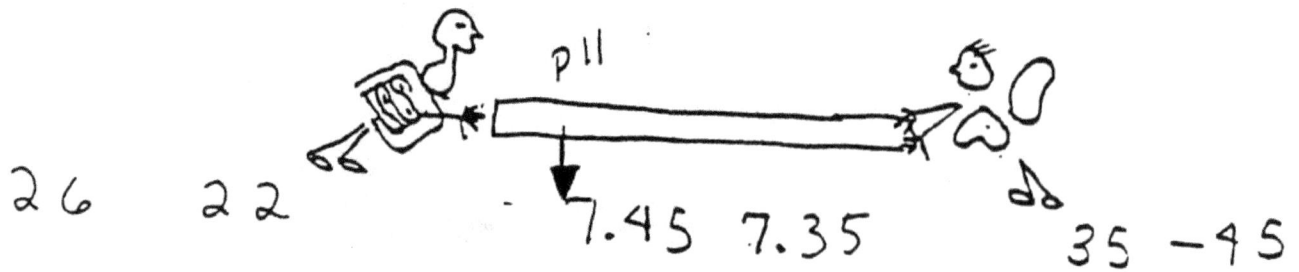

pH

26   22   7.45 7.35   35 -45

If the kidney's didn't quite get the pH past 7.45 (into normal limits) - close but not quite, that would be partial compensation.

Respiratory Compensation

Do you remember some other causes of metabolic alkalosis?

Excessive vomiting

Too many antacids

The lungs can help.......

by breathing s...l...o...w...e...r

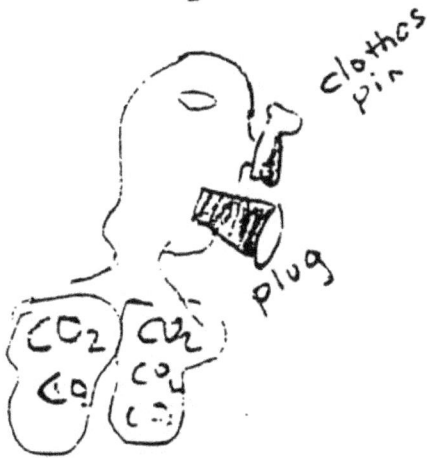

That way CO_2 piles up in the lungs. Then CO_2 piles up in the blood. Carbonic acid piles up. There is more H+ ions.

That produces more H+ than the excess bicarb can consume.

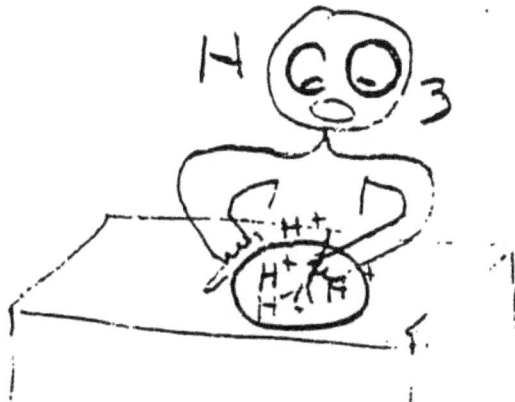

Which brings the pH closer to normal.

Metabolic alkalosis you remember looks like high bicarb pulling the pH to alkalosis

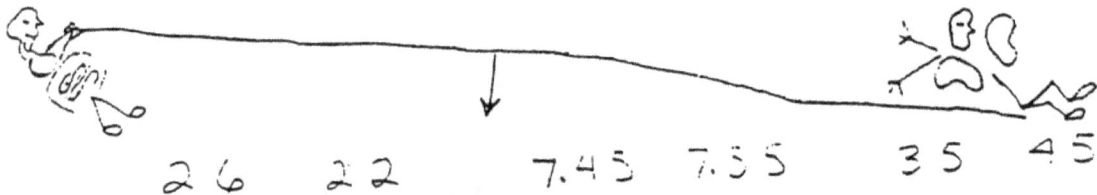

26   22   7.45 7.35   35   45

And the lungs doing nothing to stop it.

When the pH alarm goes off, the lungs spring into action or non-action by slowing the respiration rate. That lets CO_2 build up and as a result lots of H+ ions.

"phew...I did it"

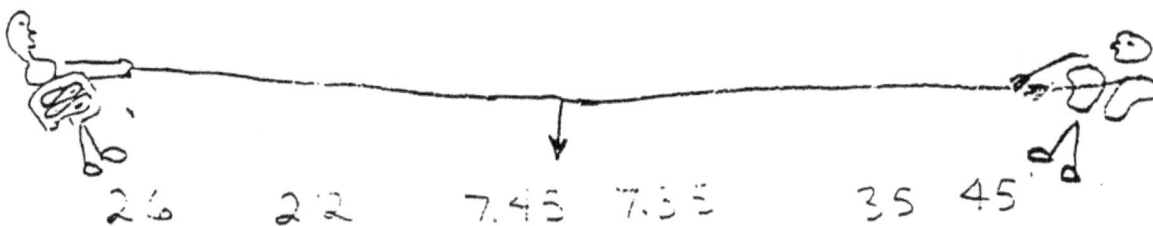

26   22   7.45 7.35   35 45

That would be metabolic alkalosis with
full respiratory compensation - a pH in
normal limits.

But is the lungs don't quite pull the pH
all the way to normal that would be
partial respiratory compensation.

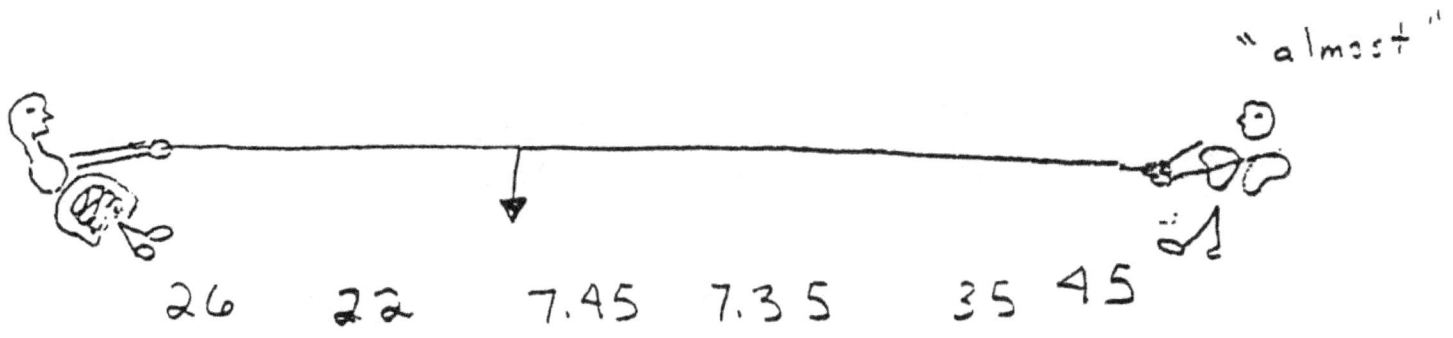

"almost"

26   22   7.45   7.35   35 45

Metabolic Acidosis With
Respiratory Compensation

You remember metabolic acidosis is caused by either a loss of bicarbonate (diarrhea) excessive acid build up (diabetic ketoacidosis or kidney failure).

The best example is Kussmaul breathing, the classic sign of diabetic ketoacidosis. This deep rapid breathing is the lungs attempt to hyperventilate out all the CO_2.

First the kidneys, intestines or metabolizing fat (diabetic ketoacidosis) throw off lots of H+ ions, that causes acidosis. This shows up on blood gases as low bicarb because all the H+ ions grab the bicarb.

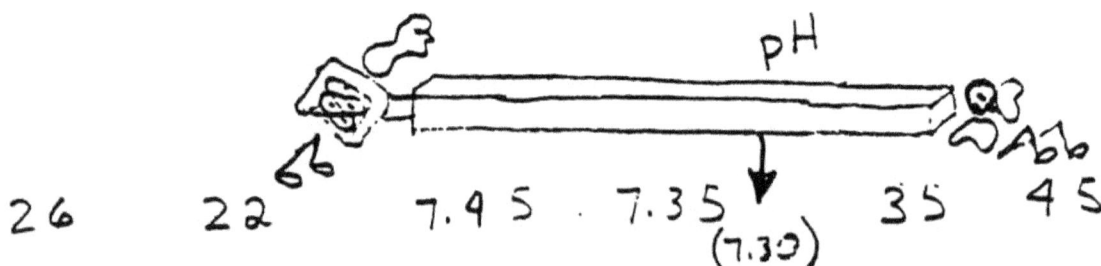

26   22   7.45   7.35   35   45
                       (7.30)

Then the lungs spring into action. They
blow off lots of CO_2 by hyperventilating.
That pulls CO_2 from
the blood and lowers
the acidity (raises
pH) very quickly.

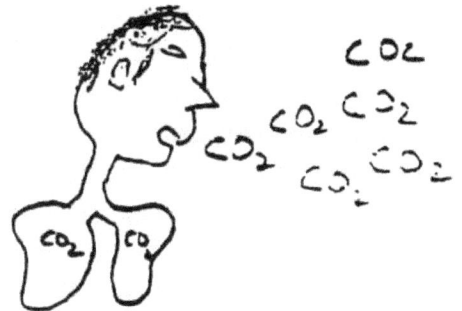

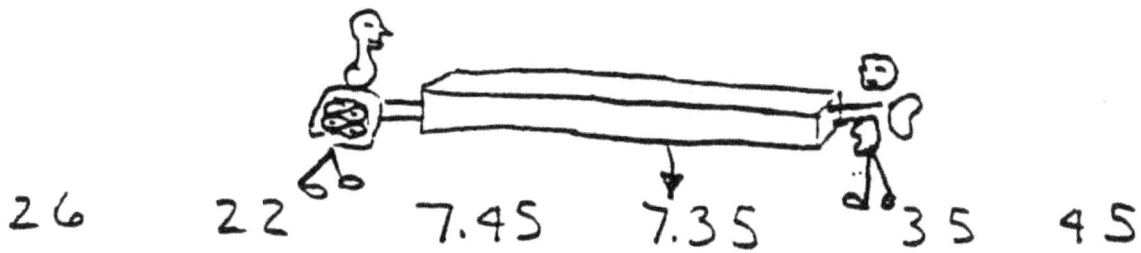

26   22   7.45   7.35   35   45

If the lungs don't quite do the job, then
it would only be partial compensation.

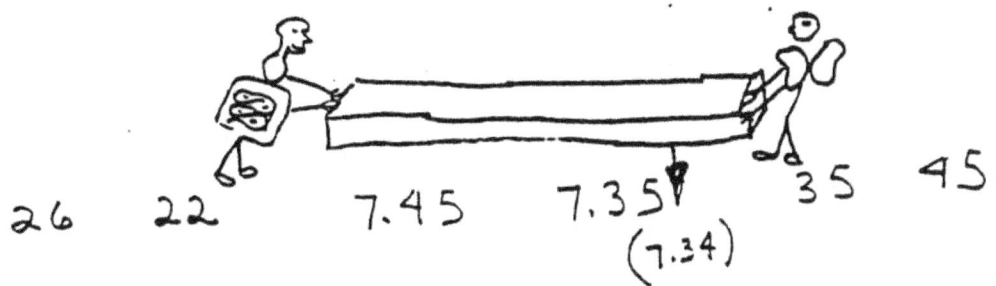

26   22   7.45   7.35   35   45
                          (7.34)

MEDICAL JOKES

Cardiac Joke: What do you get when you spill a urinal?
(see bottom of page for answer)

Immunology Joke: "I'm allergic to lasix. It makes me pee."

Hematology Joke: A vampire goes into a blood bank and asks for one unit of packed red cells and one unit of fresh frozen plasma. The phlebotomist yells back to the tech, "Gimme a Blud and a Blud Lite."

Otolaryngology Joke. For otitis media the doctor ordered "corticosporin drops in the R ear QID" The pharmacist called back to say corticosporin doesn't come in suppository form.

Orthopedic Joke (told by an infectious disease doctor): What do you need to do to pass the orthopedic boards? Be able to bench 200 pounds and spell Ancef.

Urology Joke: The doctor is doing a prostate exam. The guy yells, "That hurts!"
 The doctor says," I'm using two fingers."
"Why?"
"I want a second opinion."

Infectious Disease Joke: How do you get a Kleenex to dance? Put a little boogie in it.

 C.V. Joke: Did you hear about the two red blood cells who loved in vein?

To impress someone try saying, a gram of acetaminocin instead of two extra strength Tylenols.

G.I. Cartoon: There is a doctor, a nurse and a patient. The patient is draped and in the jack knife position presumabley for a sigmoidoscopy.. The nurse is holding a tray with a bottle of beer. The doctor with an angry look says, "No, I said I wanted a butt light."

I.C.U. Cartoon: There is a patient in an I.C.U. bed with monitors , dynamaps, oxygen, and all the familiar paraphanalia. He is talking on the phone saying, "Bells are ringing and the T.V.has a straight line."

A guy goes in to see a doctor. He touches his head and says, every time I touch it here it hurts." He touches his stomach and says the same thing. He touches his knee and repeats it again. The doctor examines him and says, "Your finger is broken."

Answer to cardiology joke: You get a Pee Wave

A very attractive young man and a vivacious young lady meet in a fashionable night club and they hit it off immediately. Later in the evening they discuss spending the night together and leave immediately for the woman's apartment. As they are getting ready for bed the woman goes into the bathroom and starts to compulsively wash her hands for an excessive length of time. The man asks, "Are you a doctor?"

"Yes."

"Don't tell me! A surgeon! Right?"

"Yes. How did you know?"

"It was obvious. I could see your concern for transmitting germs and preventing infection."

They go have sex and afterward, the woman asks the man, "Are you a doctor?"

"Yes."

"Don't tell me! An anesthesiologist! Right?"

"Yes. How did you know?"

"I didn't feel a thing."

Ophthamology Joke: This takes place in a very exclusive private girls' school. The eighth grade science teacher, Mr. Johnson, asks, " What organ of the body, when stimulated, expands to six times its normal size? Miss Smith?"

"Mr. Johnson, I don't think that is a proper question to ask a girl of my age and social standing."

He calls on another student, "Miss Jones?"

"The pupil of the eye"

"That is correct. Miss Smith I have three things to say to you. One: you didn't do your homework. Two: you have a dirty mind. Three: someday you are going to be very disappointed."

Orthopedic Joke. A guy sees a doctor. He says, "Everywhere I touch it hurts." He touches his forehead and says, "It hurts." He touches his stomach. Same thing. He touches his knee. Again, same thing. The doctor says, "Let me examine you." After a few minutes of poking and prodding, "Your finger is broken."

Ask any surgeon to name the three best surgeons in the world. They'll have a hard time thinking of the other two.

How can you tell a rectal thermometer from an oral thermometer?
For answer see bottom of the page.

A man on a crowded bus a man sees a woman with grocery bags and two small children. He gets up to give her his seat and helps her with the bags.

"Thank you. You're sweet" she says.

"I know. I'm diabetic."

Thanks to Dr. Murray Miller, an endocrinologist, for that one.

Answer to thermometer riddle: the taste.

Plastic Surgery: During routine surgery a woman goes into cardiac arrest. After superhuman efforts and being apparently dead she miraculously recovers. During this ordeal she has an out-of-body experience in which she talks to God. God tells her she has forty more years to live and she should make the most of it be striving to be her best. From that she concludes she should improve her appearance and has liposuction, breast augmentation and a face lift. As she is leaving the hospital a bus hits her and instantly kills her. When she gets to heaven she asks God," What's this all about? You said..." God interrupts, "I didn't recognize you."

Surgery: How does a surgeon change a light bulb? They Just hold it in the socket and stand still. The earth revolves around them.

Psychiatry: How many psychiatrists does it take to change a light bulb?
Only one. But first, the light bulb has to want to change.

A man on a crowded bus a man sees a woman with grocery bags and two small children. He gets up to give her his seat and helps her with the bags.
"Thank you. You're sweet" she says.
"I know. I'm diabetic."
Thanks to Dr. Murray Miller, an endocrinologist, for that one.

How do you tell the difference between an oral thermometer and a rectal thermometer? The taste.

Why did the cookie go to the doctor? It was feeling crummy.

An internist, a psychiatrist, a surgeon and a pathologist are duck hunting. The internist sees something moving in the trees. He says to the psychiatrist, "Is that a duck?" The psychiatrist says, "It's a duck if it thinks it's a duck." The surgeon grabs his shot gun, BAM BAM BAM and says to the pathologist, "Tell me if that is a duck."

Do you have any good, clean medical jokes? If you do, please send it to me. If I include it on this list, I will give you a copy of any one of my books. Also please specify whether you want your name included as the contributor – or would like to remain anonymous. Please send jokes to Malcolm Rosenberg, P.O. Box 770793, Coral Springs FL 33077 and tell me which book you want. Simplified Arterial Blood Gases, Simplified Ventilators, Simplified Hemodynamics, Drug Calculations for Nurses Who Hate Numbers, or Making the Patients Laugh.

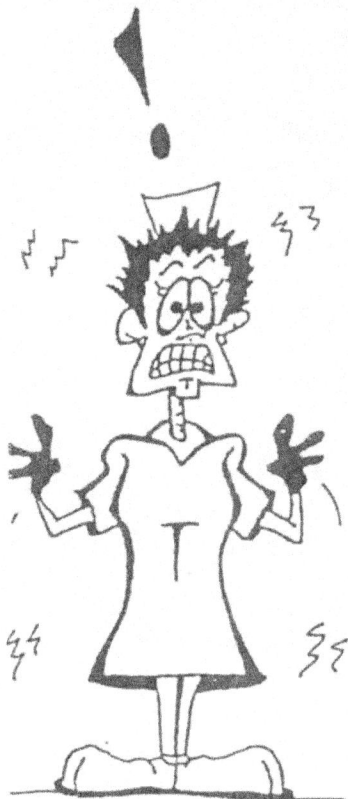
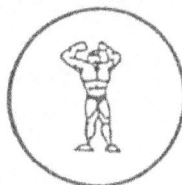 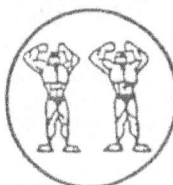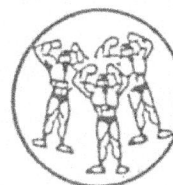
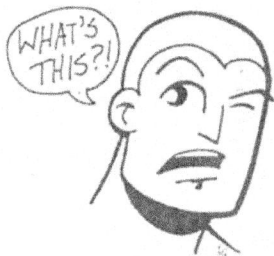

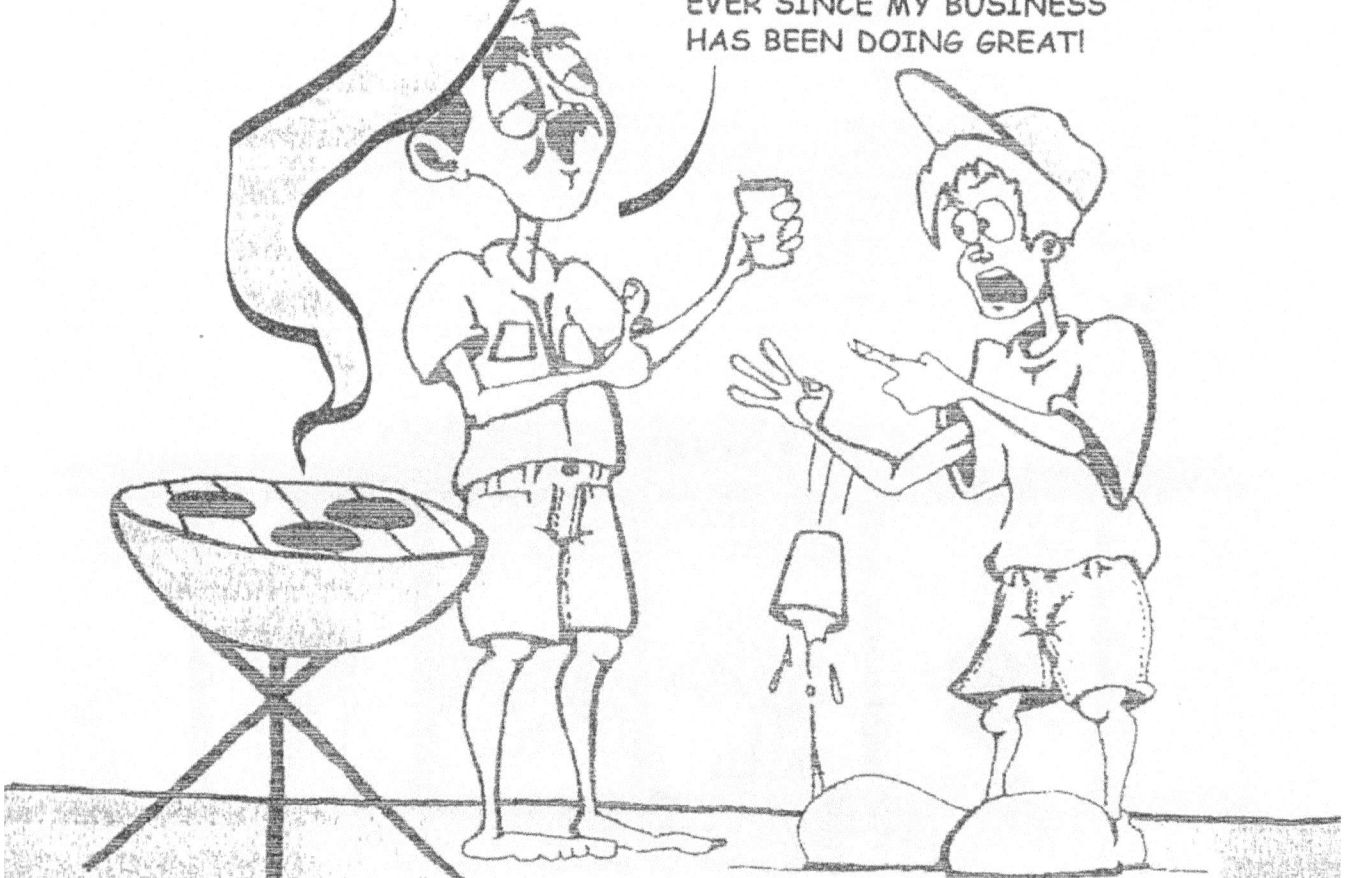

Simplified Arterial Blood Gases ©1996

Retail: $18.95

ISBN 0-9725483-1-9

9780972548311

0 700814 497996

7 00814 49799 6

www.ingramcontent.com/pod-product-compliance
Lightning Source LLC
Chambersburg PA
CBHW051223200326
41519CB00025B/7220